Rapid Revision in Clinical Pharmacology

Ben Greenstein

PhD MRPharms BA(Hons) FRIH
HONORARY SENIOR RESEARCH FELLOW
PAIN MANAGEMENT SERVICE
ROYAL FREE HOSPITAL, LONDON

Radcliffe Publishing
Oxford • New York

Radcliffe Publishing Ltd
18 Marcham Road
Abingdon
Oxon OX14 1AA
United Kingdom

www.radcliffe-oxford.com

Electronic catalogue and worldwide online ordering facility.

British Library Cataloguing in Publication Data

A catalogue record for this book is available from the British Library.

ISBN-13: 978 1 85775 795 8

Typeset by Pindar New Zealand (Egan Reid), Auckland, New Zealand
Printed and bound by TJI Digital, Padstow, Cornwall, UK

Contents

About the author

Ben Greenstein graduated as a Pharmacist in South Africa in 1965 and immigrated to the UK with his wife in 1966 where, after three years as a Community Pharmacist in London he obtained a PhD in pharmacology at Chelsea College, University of London in 1975, studying molecular aspects of steroid hormone action. After carrying out endocrine research at Oxford University for three years as a Senior Research Fellow of the Mental Health Foundation, he took a post as lecturer in the Department of Pharmacology in St Thomas' Hospital Medical School (now absorbed into King's College, London) until 1992, after which he directed an endocrine research group studying endocrine aspects of lupus in the Lupus Research Unit in St Thomas' Hospital. In 1999 he moved to the Arizona Arthritis Center in the University of Arizona in Tucson as a Senior Visiting Research Professor, and returned to the UK in 2001, where he is currently a Visiting Senior Research Fellow in the Department of Pain Management Services. He has produced textbooks of pharmacology, endocrinology and neuroscience for undergraduate students.

For Lorraine

1 Introduction

This book is intended for the student in a hurry. It was written by someone who has experienced the terror associated with realising that an examination is just around the corner. The book addresses the needs of the student who:
- at the beginning of an academic year needs a clear picture of the overall shape and size of the topic
- asks about its relevance to the ultimate aim of the field of study
- may need direction on how the information can be concisely and accessibly arranged in preparation for examination.

You will find practical suggestions for the preparation of easily accessible notes which, from personal experience, the writer has found to be useful. These suggestions are offered in the knowledge that some readers prefer a more cursive style of information storage and retrieval, but it is hoped that some may find the method presented here useful.

Approaching the task at hand

Below are some of the printable exhortations used by this writer to help him get down to revision (and to writing this book).
- No one made me get into this.
- I'm hoping this will help others.
- It's better late than never.
- At least I've got this book.
- Just think of that pass list.
- I'm as good as the others.
- This won't beat me.
- Either life's got its foot on my neck, or I've got my foot on life's neck.
- No one's going to do this for me.

Making notes for and during revision

- Ideally, notes should be made as soon as possible after a lecture when the information is still fresh in the mind. However, sometimes this is not possible. The disadvantage of not having good notes can be turned to an advantage by using note preparation as a form of revision.

- Revision notes should be as brief and concise as possible – lecture notes are usually not brief and concise.
- Heavy textbooks do not automatically transfer their contents to the buyer's brain on purchase, and some students do not have time to assimilate such books.
- Revision notes, especially in an emergency, should be portable and their information instantly accessible.

A suggested method of compiling notes for revision purposes

Equipment needed: filing cards 8 in × 5 in (20 × 13 cm) and pens, pencils and erasers. These are available from stationery shops and some supermarkets. All the information about a drug – its mechanisms, uses etc – will be written on the card. The card system can also be used for making tables, diagrams and graphs. The overriding principle is to simplify, summarise and reduce the volume of notes.

You may ask why the book does not contain finished cards. The process of producing revision cards is a powerful form of learning, so readers are encouraged to do this for themselves. A vital part of this learning method is to find the information relevant to a given heading.

Below is an example of a revision card for the drug digoxin.

Drug: digoxin **Source**: foxglove (*Digitalis lanta*); synthetic **Uses**: atrial fibrillation; atrial flutter; congestive heart failure uncontrolled by other drugs **Preparations**: oral tables 125 or 250 μg; IV in emergency **Mechanism of action**: (i) inhibition of Na^+/K^+ ATPase pump, causing raised intracellular Ca^{2+} (for treating heart failure); (ii) increasing vagal activity slowing the heart (for treating arrhythmia)	**Safety margin**: narrow therapeutic index: therapeutic plasma concentration = 0.5–1.5 ng/ml; toxic conc. = >2 ng/ml; safety margin reduced in presence of low K^+. **Symptoms of digoxin toxicity**: arrhythmias; ventricular tachycardia; disturbance of vision – yellow-green halo **Treatment of digoxin poisoning**: gastric lavage if a recent dose; antibody fragments to digoxin; some sources advocate haemodialysis **Drug interactions**: potentially dangerous with amiodarone, erythromycin, verapamil

FIGURE 1.1

There is a quiz at the end of each chapter. It follows the subject of the chapter closely and is intended as a supplement and a reminder of the chapter's contents. The questions are for the most part True/False choices and there are some gentle 'traps'. The quizzes are designed to reinforce the information presented in the chapter.

Finally, it is worth mentioning that pharmacology is not really about drugs – it is about people. When I first started teaching the subject to medical and dental students, the most frequent complaint was that the subject was not relevant. Students asked, 'Why do I have to know anything about receptors to help patients?' It took me a long time to develop the right answer, which is that pharmacology is not about drugs, it is about helping patients – helping them to feel no pain, to feel encouraged, to relieve symptoms and, if possible, to get them well again. And apart from surgery, drugs are virtually all we have when confronted by disease – apart from complementary medicine and TLC.

Author's note

Readers may notice that not much attention is paid here to hormones as drugs. This is more fully covered in the companion volume, *Rapid Revision in Endocrinology* by Ben Greenstein (Oxford: Racliffe Publishing; 2007).

Further reading

Greenstein B, Greenstein A. *Concise Clinical Pharmacology*. London: Pharmaceutical Press; 2007.

2 Pharmacology overview

Learning objectives ■ A definition of pharmacology ■ Main divisions of
pharmacology ■ Pharmacodynamics ■ Pharmacokinetics ■ Sources of
drugs ■ Relevance of pharmacology to health care ■ Pharmacokinetics
■ Pharmacoeconomics ■ The QALY – Quality Adjusted Life Year ■
Pharmacovigilance ■ Summary of systems targeted by drugs

Learning objectives
- Know the meanings of the different branches of pharmacology.
- Be able to give a definition of pharmacology.
- Have an idea of the different sources of drugs.
- Be acquainted with the terminology given here for pharmacoeconomics.
- Know what pharmacovigilance is, and briefly what it involves.

A definition of pharmacology
Pharmacology is the science of drug action on and interaction with living
systems and other organisms such as viruses.

Main divisions of pharmacology
- Pharmacodynamics.
- Pharmacokinetics.*
- Pharmacoeconomics.
- Pharmacovigilance.

- **Pharmacodynamics** is the study of how the drug affects the organism.
- **Pharmacokinetics** is the study of how the organism affects the drug.
- **Pharmacoeconomics** is the study of the cost/benefit ratio in comparison
  with other drugs or strategies aimed at a particular treatment.
- **Pharmacovigilance** is the study of the detection, assessment,
  understanding, assessment and prevention of adverse effects of medicines.

Pharmacodynamics *(see Chapter 4)*
- The receptor concept:
  - the concept of specificity – receptors for drugs
  - agonists and antagonists

---

* Pharmacokinetics is often taken to include pharmacoeconomics and pharmacovigilance, but they are
separated here for purposes of clarity and ease of learning.

- second messenger systems and genomic activation
- the measurement of drug activity
  - the dose-response curve
  - bioassay and other assay systems
  - clinical trials.

Pharmacokinetics *(see Chapter 3)*
- Basic principles of drug absorption:
  - routes of administration
  - bioavailability and membrane penetration.
- Distribution of drugs in the body.
- Metabolism of drugs.
- Excretion of drugs.

Sources of drugs
- Plant sources, e.g. Vincristine (from the periwinkle) for treatment of cancer of the lymphatic system.
- Mineral sources, e.g. calcium carbonate.
- Animal sources, e.g. vaccines.
- Synthetic, e.g. temazepam, a short-acting hypnotic (for sleep).
- Biosynthetic, e.g. recombinant proteins such as the TNF-α antibody for rheumatoid arthritis (*see* p. 73).

Relevance of pharmacology to health care
- Pharmacology 'Need to know' now applies to:[*]
  - doctors
  - pharmacists
  - nurses
  - dentists
  - practitioners of complementary medicine.

Pharmacokinetics
Pharmacokinetics is the scientific study of how the body processes the drug, i.e. what the body does with the drug. It deals with:
- absorption of the drug
- distribution of the drug in the different body compartments
- metabolism of the drug
- excretion of the drug
- half-life of the drug, i.e. the time taken for half the amount of the drug or other substance to be metabolised or eliminated

---

[*] These days this can never be comprehensive, for example supermarkets sell drugs.

- toxicity of the drug
- formulation of the drug for administration, based on the knowledge obtained
- clinical trials in drug development prior to licensing for general clinical use.

Pharmacoeconomics*

Pharmacoeconomics is the comparison of ratios of:
- cost/benefit – this is the comparison of relative costs of two or more treatments which treat the same problem
- cost-effectiveness – this is the comparison of different treatments in order to decide which will give best value for money in terms of symptom reduction, chance of a cure, or best chance of reducing the risks of mortality from the problem being treated (for example)
- cost-minimisation – this is the comparison of the costs of different treatments when all give the same effectiveness (a relatively rare situation)
- cost utility – this is the comparison of different treatments in terms of their contribution to the patient's increased quality of life (*see* QALY below).

Note: these parameters refer not only to comparisons between different drugs but sometimes also between drugs or other options, e.g. surgery.

The QALY – Quality Adjusted Life Year

The QALY is used to relate health to money and to decide which patients should get treatment.
- The QALY can have a value between 0 and 1.
- QALY = 1 means one year with no illness after treatment.
- QALY = 0 means death (although some might say that some life qualities, e.g. total immobilisation, are worse than death).
- The closer the value is to 1, the better the health gain after treatment.
- Obviously you don't know the value for a given patient until after treatment, but it may have usefulness as a predictor.

Pharmacovigilance

Pharmacovigilance is the study of the detection, measurement or assessment of adverse reactions, both in the short and long term.
- Involves the collection and evaluation of the adverse effects of treatment, mainly of drug-related treatments.
- Aims to assess and reduce the risks associated with the taking of medicines

---

* Also called outcomes research and a sore subject in some quarters; this is an extremely abridged treatment.

or use of other forms of medical intervention (risk management).

- Measures risks by comparing benefits with adverse effects. For example, bisphosphonates are widely used and powerful protective agents against osteoporosis (bone thinning and fracture), but can, if not taken properly cause potentially dangerous oesophageal damage through reflux.
- Operates through:
  - local and international monitoring and regulatory bodies, e.g. the WHO International Drug Monitoring Programme, the US Food and Drug Administration (FDA), the European Medicines Agency and the British Committee on Safety of Medicines
  - spontaneous reporting by health practitioners
  - reports by manufacturers
  - reports from clinical trials
  - reports by pharmacists and nurses
  - last but not least, reports by patients.

Summary of systems targeted by drugs

- Autonomic nervous system.
- Blood.
- Cardiovascular system.
- Central nervous system.
- Digestive system.
- Endocrine and exocrine systems.
- Immune system.
- Senses.
- Skin.
- Urogenital systems.

3 Pharmacokinetics

Learning objectives ■ Pharmacokinetics ■ Drug absorption ■ Drug distribution ■ Drug metabolism ■ Drug excretion

Learning objectives

- Know the routes of administration of drugs.
- Know what the choice of route depends on.
- Be able to list the body compartments given.
- Be acquainted with the concept of the volume of distribution.
- Know what the partition coefficient is.
- Be able to give a brief account of the significance of plasma binding of drugs.
- Be able to give a brief account of the principles of drug metabolism.
- Know the routes of drug excretion and how excretion is measured.

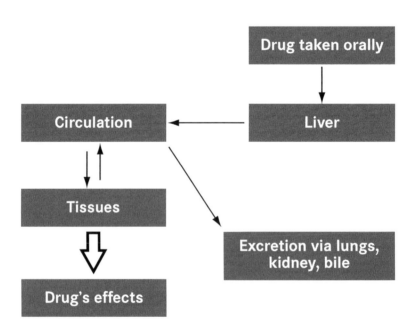

FIGURE 3.1 Pathways of drugs which act systemically.

Pharmacokinetics

Pharmacokinetics is the scientific study of how the body processes the drug, i.e. what the body does with the drug. It deals with:

- absorption of the drug
- distribution of the drug in the different body compartments
- metabolism of the drug
- excretion of the drug
- half-life of the drug, i.e. the time taken for half the amount of the drug or other substance to be metabolised or eliminated
- toxicity of the drug
- formulation of the drug for administration, based on the knowledge obtained
- clinical trials, which are the final steps in drug development prior to licensing for general clinical use.

Drug absorption

External environment
e.g. lumen of GIT

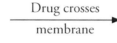

Drug crosses
membrane

Internal environment
e.g. into bloodstream,
cell, extracellular fluid

- Routes of administration:
  - oral, e.g. paracetamol
  - sublingual, e.g. glyceryl trinitrate for angina
  - parenteral (injection), e.g. insulin for diabetes
  - inhalation, e.g. salbutamol
  - rectal, e.g. corticosteroids for haemorrhoids
  - vaginal, e.g. clotrimazole for candidiasis
  - topical, e.g. fluocinonide cream for eczema
  - inhalation, e.g. general anaesthetics
  - transdermal, e.g. long-acting steroids.
- Choice of route depends on:
  - the site of action required
  - patient convenience; the oral route is the most convenient and least stressful way of taking drugs that need to be absorbed into the internal environment
  - speed of onset required; IV gives the most rapid onset, e.g. in emergencies, (status asthmaticus)
  - limitations for absorption; uncharged molecules, e.g. steroids are absorbed more rapidly than charged molecules such as aspirin; some drugs are destroyed in the gut, such as insulin, which has to be administered parentally or by inhalation

- duration of drug action, e.g. SC implants of steroids may last months, removing the need to remember to take timed doses
- organ exclusion, e.g. modern antihistamines are designed not to cross the blood–brain barrier appreciably, which reduces drowsiness
- localisation requirements, e.g. local anaesthetics are applied topically in order to reduce access to the circulation, which could be dangerous, since local anaesthetics can cause fatal arrhythmias.

Drug distribution

Body compartment can be thought of as:
- extracellular water ± 0.2 l/kg
- intracellular water
- bone ± 0.75 l/kg.
- vascular water ± 0.4 l/kg
- fat ± 0.3 l/kg

The distribution of a drug depends on its properties, mainly:
- solubility in water
- degree of ionisation
- lipid solubility
- molecular weight.

The volume of distribution (V_D)
- Is a theoretical measurement that has been designed to try and measure the distribution of the drug between various compartments.
- Can be thought of as the volume of water that the body would need to have so that the extravascular concentration of the drug would be the same as that in plasma.
- Is useful since it gives an idea about how available the drug is for treatment, e.g. the higher the V_D the more likely it is that the drug is tucked away from the bloodstream, e.g. dissolved in fat and therefore is not available to the tissue that needs the drug.
- Gives an indication of dose required; the higher the V_D, the higher the loading dose may need to be.
- Is calculated using this formula:

$$V_D = \frac{\text{amount of drug in body}}{\text{plasma concentration}}$$

Note: the V_D is a purely theoretical concept; it is a ratio and is not the measurement of a volume.

The partition coefficient
- Is a ratio of the distribution of a drug between two different phases, e.g. water and oil; the potency of general anaesthetics is positively correlated with the oil:water coefficient of the general anaesthetic.

Plasma proteins
- Bind drugs (and some circulating hormones), which affects their distribution and availability to the tissues.
- There is an equilibrium between bound and unbound (free) drug in plasma.
- Only the unbound drug (often < 5% of the total) is available to the tissues.
- Examples of plasma drug-binding proteins:
  - albumin – binds many drugs
  - sex hormone-binding globulin – binds estradiol and testosterone
  - thyroxine-binding globulin – binds thyroid hormone.
- This may cause unwanted drug effects; some drugs displace others and may increase unbound concentrations of a drug to overdose levels, e.g. clofibrate displaces warfarin from plasma proteins, thus raising free warfarin concentrations in plasma, which could be dangerous.

Drug metabolism
- The major site of drug metabolism is the liver.
- First pass metabolism of drugs. All drugs taken orally into the GIT are absorbed into the mesenteric veins, which drain into the portal vein and then into the liver. In the liver much of the drug may be metabolised. This results in the reduction in the efficacy of a single dose, which will need to be increased, or an alternative dosage route used.
- Drug metabolism is classified as:
  - Phase I reactions, which change the structure of the drug, often to render it polar and therefore more soluble, e.g. through hydrolysis or oxidation-reduction reactions
  - Phase II reactions, which combine the Phase 1-modified drug with a conjugate, e.g. glucuronide, sulphate, methyl group or by acetylation.
- Consequences of drug metabolism may be:
  - drug inactivation, e.g. demethylation of morphine (about 5%)
  - drug activation, e.g. demethylation of inactive imipramine to active desipramine, an antidepressant
  - to render drugs easier to excrete by making them more water-soluble, e.g. metabolism of morphine to morphine glucuronide (95%).

A warning note: some drugs can become lethal when metabolised, e.g. paracetamol in safe doses is conjugated mainly to a glucuronide or sulphate and ± 5% is conjugated to glutathione. At more than double the recommended therapeutic dose (0.5–1 gram every 4–6 hours to a maximum of 4 grams every 24 hours) glutathione stores may be depleted and excess paracetamol is metabolised to potentially hepatotoxic products.

The degree of drug metabolism depends not only on the nature of the drug, but also on:

■ what other drugs are being taken, including alcohol or cigarette smoke
■ the patient's age
■ the patient's state of health, especially liver function
■ genetic factors.

Drug excretion

Drugs may be excreted from the body via:

■ faeces
■ lungs
■ milk
■ saliva
■ sweat
■ urine (for most drugs in use).

Excretion usually occurs via two or more of these routes, the relative contribution depending on the nature of the drug.

The rate of excretion of drugs needs to be known and is measured using:

■ glomerular filtration rate
■ plasma and urine concentrations
■ the drug's clearance
■ the half-life ($t\frac{1}{2}$) of the drug in plasma
■ the volume of distribution (V_D)
■ the kinetics of elimination of a drug may be:
  ❚ First order, which means that the rate of elimination of the drug is related to the concentration of the drug in plasma. The higher the

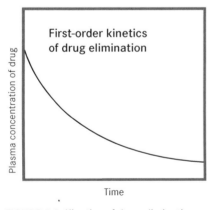
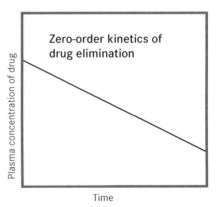

FIGURE 3.2 Kinetics of drug elimination.

concentrations, the faster it is excreted. This is a sensible strategy and safer for the body, which wants to get the levels of a foreign chemical down fast (*see* Figure 3.2)

- Zero order, which means that the rate of elimination is the same no matter what the concentration of the drug in plasma. This is potentially dangerous, especially in cases of over-dosage, e.g. with alcohol.

Chapter 3 Quiz

ANSWER T (TRUE) OR F (FALSE)

1. Subcutaneous injection gives the most rapid onset of drug action. ☐ F
2. Uncharged molecules are absorbed more rapidly after oral administration. ☐ T
3. Drug distribution is independent of its lipid solubility. ☐ F
4. The higher the volume of distribution, the higher the dose that may be needed. ☐ T
5. The plasma protein-bound drug is the form available to the tissues. ☐ F
6. The major site of drug metabolism is the liver. ☐ T
7. First pass metabolism can reduce the efficacy of a drug. ☐ T
8. Phase I reactions conjugate the drug (e.g.) to a glucuronide. ☐ F
9. Metabolism is the invariable method for inactivating drugs. ☐ F
10. Drugs are easier for the body to excrete when rendered more soluble. ☐ T
11. Genetic factors can affect the degree of drug metabolism. ☐ T
12. Most drugs are excreted via the faeces. ☐ F
13. Measurement of drug half-life is not used to measure the rate of drug excretion. ☐ F
14. First order kinetics means that the rate of drug excretion is faster when plasma concentrations of the drug are higher. ☐ T

4 Pharmacodynamics

Learning objectives

■ Know what the term 'receptor' means in pharmacological terms.
■ Be able to explain the receptor properties of affinity, selectivity and reversibility.
■ Know the difference between drug potency and drug efficacy.
■ Be able to draw the dose-response and $\log_{10}$ dose-response curves and explain how drug potencies and receptor antagonists are graphically portrayed on the $\log_{10}$ dose-response curve.
■ Know what is meant by antagonists and their properties.
■ Be familiar with the concept of signal transduction in relation to pharmacodynamics.
■ Be able to list some important second messenger systems.

Pharmacodynamics

Pharmacodynamics is the scientific study of:
■ how the drug signals to its target cells that it is there (receptors)
■ how the cell can tell the difference between different drugs (specificity)
■ the reaction between the drug and the cell's drug recognition mechanism (i.e. the receptor)
■ how to gauge the potency, specificity and efficacy of the drug
■ the mechanisms through which the cell produces its response to the drug (e.g. second messenger systems; transcriptional changes)
■ how to use this information to design better, safer and more specific drugs
■ how the drug affects the body, as opposed to pharmacokinetics, which is about how the body affects the drug.

The receptor*

■ Is a protein, either on the cell's surface (e.g. the epinephrine receptor) or inside the cell (e.g. the estrogen receptor).

---

* The term 'receptor' is used also in the study of the senses to describe the organ that transduces sensory inputs, for example touch into an action potential.

- Has properties of selectivity and high affinity for the drug.
- Is often there because the body has endogenous ligands* for the receptor (e.g. the body possesses endogenous opioids which bind the receptors for morphine).
- Is a frequent target of drug designers.
- Is designed according to its location and function (for example):
  - extracellular receptors have extracellular, intramembrane and intracellular domains, and bind to drugs and endogenous chemicals that (usually) do not penetrate the cell
  - intracellular receptors are inside the cell and bind to drugs and endogenous chemicals (e.g. steroids) that penetrate the cell membrane.

Receptor properties important in pharmacology
- Affinity.
- Selectivity.
- Reversibility of ligand binding.

Receptor affinity describes how powerful the attraction between drug, hormone etc and the receptor is. In theory, the higher the potency of the drug, the lower the dose needed.

Receptor selectivity describes the ability of the receptor to distinguish between drugs so that some are bound and others not. In pharmacological terms, this is conceivably the most important principle of chemical reactions with tissues.

Reversibility of ligand binding means that the chemical, e.g. drug or hormone, is able to dissociate from the receptor, usually leaving both chemical and receptor physically and chemically unchanged.

Drug potency and efficacy
- The potency of a drug can be defined as the relationship between the dose and the magnitude of the desired effect, and is most conveniently assessed using the dose-response curve (*see* below and Figure 4.1a).
- Drug efficacy is often confused with drug potency. Efficacy describes how efficient a given dose of drug is in the body. One drug may have a higher measurable potency than another using *in vitro*† tests, but produce a lesser therapeutic effect if it is more quickly metabolised.

---

* Ligand: the term for a chemical that binds to another chemical; in pharmacology this usually refers to a drug.
† *In vitro*: within the glass, for example in the test tube.

The dose-response curve

- Is obtained by measuring a given parameter (e.g. blood pressure fall) in response to a range of doses of the test drug.
- Gives an approximate idea of the potency of the drug in terms of the dose which gives the maximum response.
- Is converted to the log_{10} dose-response curve to give a linear segment more amenable to calculation (*see* Figure 4.1b) in that:
  - the log_{10} dose-response curve can be used to compare the relative potency of two or more drugs on a given parameter[*] (*see* Figure 4.1c)
  - it can be used to test the potency of an antagonist drug (*see* Figure 4.1d).

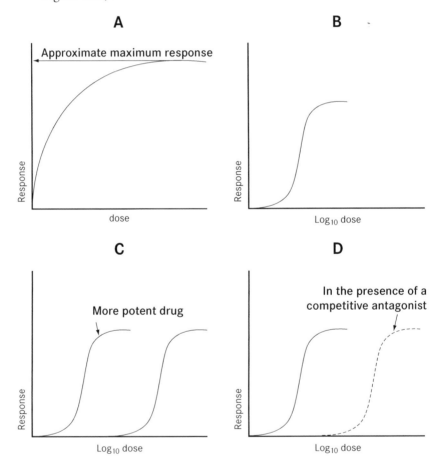

A

Approximate maximum response

Response

dose

B

Response

Log_{10} dose

C

More potent drug

Response

Log_{10} dose

D

In the presence of a competitive antagonist

Response

Log_{10} dose

FIGURE 4.1 The dose-response and log_{10} dose-response curves.

---

[*] Parameter: the variable, for example blood pressure.

Nomenclature note: an agonist is a drug that produces a response normally produced by the body's own mediator, e.g. bronchodilation produced by the drug terbutaline acting on β_2-adrenoceptors normally activated by epinephrine and norepinephrine.

A β-blocker (the antagonist) blocks the normal response by binding to β_2-adrenoceptors and blocking access to epinephrine and norepinephrine. This makes β-blockers potentially fatal in asthmatics.

Drug antagonists

- Are drugs that are recognised by a tissue but block the effect of another drug by interfering with that drug's interaction with the cell.
- May act by:
  - binding to the receptor, thus blocking access to an agonist
  - blocking a transmembrane ion channel (e.g. *see* p. 23)
  - blocking normal transcription of the DNA (e.g. *see* p. 24).
- May be used to block effects caused by the body's own chemical mediators, e.g. atropine-like drugs block parasympathetic nervous drive to the eye to dilate the pupil for eye examination (*see* p. 35).
- May be:
  - competitive, which means that increasing agonist concentration displaces antagonist from the receptor, e.g. morphine and naloxone (*see* p. 192)*
  - non-competitive, which means increasing agonist dose does not displace antagonist from the receptor
  - reversible, which means the response to agonist can be rescued by increasing agonist concentrations at the receptor site
  - irreversible, which means the antagonist cannot be displaced from the receptor, and normal resumption of function must await synthesis of more receptors, e.g. organophosphate poisoning (*see* p. 36).

Signal transduction

- Is conversion of one energy form into another, e.g. conversion of a physical binding of a chemical to a receptor into (for example):
  - an enzyme-catalysed chemical reaction
  - an electrical impulse
  - a conformational change in a protein, e.g. the receptor itself.
- May occur as a result of drug action either through agonist or antagonist action.

---

* An important principle in toxicology.

Second messenger systems

- Are (usually) intracellular systems activated or blocked by the initial drug-receptor interaction.
- When activated ultimately express the action of the endogenous or exogenous agonist.
- Include:
  - the adenylate cyclase-cyclic AMP system
  - the IP3 (Inositol triphosphate-PLC*) system
  - kinase-linked receptor systems, e.g. the insulin receptor.
- When activated may result in genomic changes, e.g. transcriptional activation or repression.

Chapter 4 Quiz

ANSWER T (TRUE) OR F (FALSE)

1. Pharmacodynamics:

   Is the study of how the body processes the drug ☐

   Includes the study of receptor dynamics ☐

   Attempts to explain the cell's response to the drug. ☐ ☐

2. The receptor:

   Is the cell's mechanism for recognising the drug ☐

   Is always situated on the membrane of the cell ☐

   Has properties of high affinity binding and selectivity ☐

   Can bind only one ligand. ☐ ☐

3. The dose-response curve:

   Describes the relationship between dose and tissue response ☐

   Is useful because it has a linear segment ☐

   Gives an approximate idea of the potency of a drug ☐

   Gives the drug dose above which there is no further increase in response. ☐ ☐

4. The $\log_{10}$ dose-response curve:

   Can be used to compare drug potencies for a given parameter ☐

   Can be used to measure the potency of a drug antagonist. ☐

5. An agonist is a drug that produces a response similar to that produced by an endogenous mediator. ☐

---

* PLC: Phospholipase C.

6. An antagonist:

Blocks the action of an agonist ☐

May act by:

a. Interfering with the metabolism of the agonist ☐

b. Competing with the agonist at its receptor site ☐

c. Blocking an ion channel in the cell membrane ☐

d. Blocking downstream events, e.g. transcription. ☐

7. An antagonist's action:

Cannot be reversed ☐

May be competitive and reversible ☐

May be irreversible and non-competitive. ☐

5 Clinical trials

Learning objectives
- Understand the aims of clinical trials and the basic statutory requirements generally stipulated for the design of clinical trials.
- Be familiar with the terms which describe the aims and set-up of the clinical trial.
- Know the primary aims of the four different phases of the clinical trial.

Clinical trials
- Are the culmination of all the preliminary experimental pharmacokinetic and pharmacodynamic studies of a treatment, which has been deemed ready for testing in humans.
- Evaluate:
  - new drugs
  - new 'me too' drugs, e.g. new β-blockers, antihistamines etc
  - new surgical and medical devices, e.g. new contraceptive devices
  - whether a new treatment is an improvement on existing treatments
  - by comparison, two similar treatments for a given medical problem.
- Are legal requirements for new surgical or medical interventions in people.
- Must be carried out under strictly controlled conditions.
- Must obtain the prior full and informed consent of participating patients or healthy volunteers.
- Must be supervised by regulatory authorities such as the European Medicines Agency, from whom approval must be obtained before a treatment may be put on the market.

The clinical trial design
- Aims to provide an objective, accurate and unbiased result.
- Aims to establish whether or not there is a causal relationship between the treatment and the human subject's reaction to the treatment.
- May be single-centre or multi-centre.

A clinical trial may be set up to carry out:[*]

- a randomised, controlled trial (RCT) of a treatment: a scientific experiment in which selected volunteers are randomly assigned to groups, one of which receives the test treatment, e.g. a new drug, and the other receives a placebo or another drug. Ideally, subjects and researchers are unaware which treatment is assigned to each group ('double-blind'). Following the treatment, patients are observed over time (prospectively). This type of study might be a cross-over trial, when after the first phase, treatments are swapped between the two groups
- a cohort study: following up prospectively the outcome for patients who have and have not already been on a treatment. This is a good way to assess short- and longer-term risks associated with the treatment being tested
- a case-control study: a retrospective study, i.e. it looks back over the history of patients who have or have not been exposed to a treatment or a health risk. This is a useful study when a prospective study might take too long, and also in cases of rare diseases, when not enough patients might be available for a prospective study
- a case report: a report on a single patient, often reporting an unexpected reaction.

Phases of a clinical trial

- Phase I: the treatment is tested on (usually) a group of healthy volunteers[†] (~25–75 volunteers) to assess the pharmacokinetics, pharmacodynamics and safety; major considerations are dose and dose frequency. There are two main types:
  - single ascending dose (SAD): test to find the maximum tolerated dose (MTD), when doses are ramped up with successive small groups of volunteers until unacceptable adverse effects appear
  - multiple ascending dose (MAD): to assess the pharmacodynamics and kinetics of the drug, e.g. $t_{1/2}$, absorption, metabolism, excretion and mechanism of action of the drug, dose-response relationships etc.
- Phase II: for treatments that pass Phase I; the drug is tested on much larger groups of volunteers and patients to test the clinical efficacy and further tests of drug toxicity and adverse effects. This is the phase when drugs are most likely to fail.
- Phase III: when drugs go through randomised, double-blind controlled clinical trials, sometimes on huge multi-centre groups of patients, following which the formal submission documents are prepared for the

---

[*] Not a comprehensive list.
[†] For some drugs, for example to treat metastatic cancer or AIDS, patients at an advanced stage of disease may be treated in Phase I.

approval of, for example, the European Medicines Agency or the US Food and Drug Administration (FDA); at least two such trials are commonly expected before approval is given (or not). While approval is pending, drugs may continue to be assessed for other possible therapeutic uses.

- Phase IV: clinical trials for follow-up after the treatment is available for general use, involving monitoring of drug safety, adverse effects and unacceptable risks to health and life. Phase IV trials may be demanded by regulatory bodies or voluntarily carried out by the company that launched the drug.

6 Receptors

Learning objectives

- Be able to define a receptor in the pharmacological context.
- Know the three main cellular locations of receptors.
- Be ready to give examples of ionotropic and metabotropic receptors.

Receptors in pharmacology*

A receptor is a cellular protein that binds selectively and with high affinity to another, usually smaller, chemical, e.g. a hormone, neurotransmitter or drug (usually called a ligand) as the first step in the cell's recognition of and ultimate response to the ligand.

- Physical location of the receptor:
  - extracellular on the cell membrane, e.g. ligand-gated ion channels
  - transmembrane: spanning the cell membrane and an integral part of it, e.g. neurotransmitter receptors, opioid receptors, insulin receptors and many more (*see* Figure 6.1a)
  - intracellular receptors (*see* Figure 6.1b), e.g. lipid-soluble steroid hormone receptors, vitamin D receptors, thyroid hormone receptors.

Ionotropic receptors (Ligand†-gated ion channels)

- Consist of:
  - an extracellular ligand-binding site
  - a transmembrane pore or ion channel usually specific for one ion, e.g. Na^+, Cl^-, K^+ or Ca^{2+}.
- Convert ligand binding into ion channel opening and a rapid (within milliseconds) cellular response, e.g. generation of a propagated action potential in a postsynaptic neurone.
- Have been classified as four receptor superfamilies:
  - ATP-gated channels, e.g. the P2X receptor, which mediates pain

---

* In physiology, receptors are sensory mechanisms for reception of inputs, for example touch, and for transduction of the input into electrical impulses.
† Note: voltage-gated ion channels open in response to changes in membrane potential rather than to ligand binding.

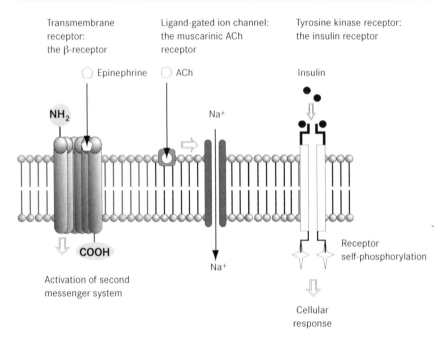

FIGURE 6.1A Cell membrane-bound receptors.

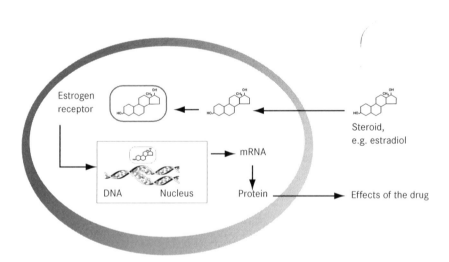

FIGURE 6.1B Intracellular steroid receptors.

▮ Cys-loop receptors, e.g. nicotinic ACh receptor
▮ glutamate receptors
▮ TRP* channels, e.g. TRPV6, a membrane-bound Ca^{2+} channel in the gastrointestinal tract.
▨ May mediate actions of drugs including CNS depressants, e.g. anaesthetics.
▨ Include:
  ▮ 5-HT$_3$ receptors
  ▮ GABA$_A$ and GABA$_C$ receptors
  ▮ glutamate receptors
  ▮ glycine receptors
  ▮ nicotinic ACh receptor.

Metabotropic receptors

▨ Are monomeric† proteins that span the cell membrane.
▨ Have seven transmembrane domains.
▨ The N-terminal of the protein is extracellular and the C-terminal is intracellular.
▨ When activated by ligands (e.g. a neurotransmitter) may:
  ▮ close or open ion channels
  ▮ activate intracellular second messenger systems, e.g. cyclic AMP or IP3
  ▮ can be classified as:
    ◆ G protein-coupled receptors: adrenoceptors, GABA$_B$ receptors, dopamine receptors, histamine receptors, opioid (e.g. morphine) receptors, somatostatin receptors
    ◆ tyrosine kinases: IGF-1 receptor, erythropoietin receptors, insulin receptors.

Second messengers

▨ Are so-called because they are the intracellular molecules that initiate the cellular response to a ligand, e.g. drug, growth factor or hormone after it has bound to a receptor on the cell membrane.
▨ Are a means of amplifying the ligand signal to the cell, e.g. the binding of one molecule of epinephrine to a β-receptor will result in the generation of several molecules of cyclic AMP.
▨ May be lipophilic and operate within the membrane environment, e.g. diacylglycerol; hydrophilic, e.g. Ca^{2+} and cyclic AMP, which operate within the cytosolic‡ compartment; gases, e.g. nitric oxide.

---

* TRP: transient receptor potential.
† Monomeric: a single molecular unit (by combining with others of the same forms a polymer).
‡ The cytosol is the extranuclear solution of water-soluble constituents.

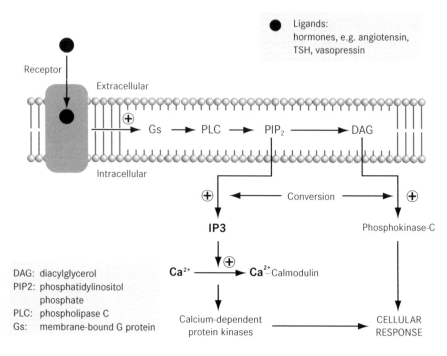

FIGURE 6.2 Inositol phosphate–PLC system (highly simplified).

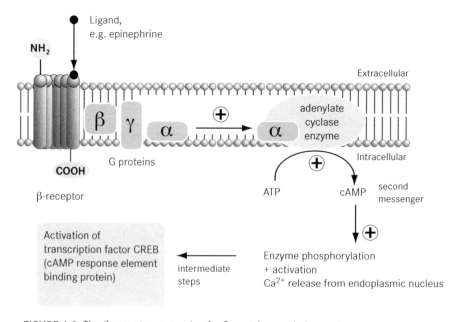

FIGURE 6.3 The β-receptor: example of a G protein–coupled receptor.

Important, known second messenger systems

- Inositol phosphate-diacylglycerol system (*see* Figure 6.2).
- Adenylate cyclase-cyclic AMP system (*see* Figure 6.3).
- Cyclic GMP system.
- Ca^{2+} system.
- Nitric oxide (NO) system.

Chapter 6 Quiz

ANSWER T (TRUE) OR F (FALSE)

1. The receptor:

   Is a protein able to recognise only one ligand. ☐

   Binds ligands with high affinity and selectivity. ☐

   May be part of the cell membrane or occur intracellularly. ☐

   Is the first step in the cell's recognition of extracellular ligands. ☐

2. Ligand-gated ion channels:

   Consist of a ligand-binding site linked to an ion pore. ☐

   Mediate long-delay transduction. ☐

   Control ATP-gated channels. ☐

   Mediate muscarinic ACh cellular responses. ☐

3. Metabotropic receptors:

   Span cell membranes with 7 transmembrane domains. ☐

   Have intracellular NH_2 terminals. ☐

   May activate intracellular second messenger systems. ☐

   Include the insulin receptor. ☐

4. Second messengers:

   Are so-called because they initiate intracellular responses to drugs. ☐

   Are a means of amplifying cellular responses to a single drug molecule. ☐

   Include cyclic AMP and diacylglycerol. ☐

7 The autonomic system I: introduction

Learning objectives ■ The autonomic nervous system ■ Autonomic nervous system structure ■ Neurotransmitters and receptors of the efferent autonomic system

Learning objectives
- Be able to list systems which are regulated by the autonomic nervous system.
- Be able to draw and label the layout of the autonomic nervous system as given below.
- Know the identities of the main neurotransmitters and receptors of the efferent division of the autonomic nervous system.

The autonomic nervous system (ANS)
- Is a division of the nervous system which is not under conscious control, i.e. involves involuntary processes.
- Controls vital systems, including:
  - the cardiovascular system
  - digestive system
  - genitourinary system
  - the respiratory system
  - smooth muscle function
  - glandular function, both endocrine and exocrine
  - the five senses
  - body temperature control.
- Consists of two main divisions that counterbalance each other functionally:
  - the parasympathetic nervous system
  - the sympathetic nervous system.
- Is an important target for therapeutic drug action.

Note: Some texts mention an enteric nervous system. This is the largely self-contained innervation of the gut.

Autonomic nervous system structure
- Control nuclei are in the CNS.

- Efferent preganglionic fibres run to relay ganglia.
- Efferent postganglionic fibres run to end organs and tissues.
- Afferent fibres run from target organs and tissues to the CNS.
- Efferent parasympathetic preganglionic fibres are generally long.
- And efferent parasympathetic postganglionic fibres are generally on the target tissue.
- Efferent sympathetic preganglionic fibres are generally short.
- And efferent sympathetic postganglionic fibres are generally long.

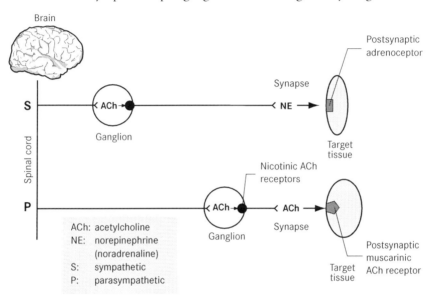

FIGURE 7.1 Diagrammatic autonomic nervous system overview.

Neurotransmitters and receptors of the efferent autonomic system

- In both sympathetic and parasympathetic divisions of the ANS, acetylcholine (ACh) is released from presynaptic preganglionic fibres and binds to postsynaptic nicotinic* receptors of postganglionic fibres.
- In the sympathetic division of the ANS, (generally) *long* postganglionic fibres terminate at the target organ and release the catecholamine norepinephrine (noradrenaline), which binds to postsynaptic adrenoceptors.
- In the parasympathetic division of the ANS, (generally) *short* postganglionic fibres terminate at the target organ and release ACh, which binds to postsynaptic muscarinic† ACh receptors.

---

* So named because they were first discovered through the use of nicotine.
† So named because they were first discovered through the use of the toadstool poison muscarine.

Chapter 7 Quiz

ANSWER T (TRUE) OR F (FALSE)

1. The autonomic nervous system controls voluntary movement. ☐ F
2. The ANS consists of sympathetic and parasympathetic divisions. ☐ T
3. Afferent preganglionic fibres carry impulses to the target organs. ☐ F
4. Efferent parasympathetic, preganglionic fibres are generally long. ☐ T
5. Afferent nerve fibres carry impulses from the CNS to the periphery. ☐ F
6. ACh is released from presynaptic, preganglionic fibres in the ganglia. ☐ T
7. ACh binds to postsynaptic nicotinic receptors in the ganglia. ☐ T
8. ACh binds to postganglionic, postsynaptic adrenoceptors on target organs. ☐ F
9. Epinephrine is the major postganglionic neurotransmitter of the sympathetic division of the ANS. ☐ F

8 The autonomic system II: parasympathetic division (PNS)

Learning objectives ■ The parasympathetic division of the ANS ■ Anatomical layout of the PNS ■ Actions of the PNS on tissues ■ Biosynthesis and metabolism of acetylcholine ■ Receptors for acetylcholine ■ Ganglionic muscarinic ACh receptors ■ Postganglionic muscarinic ACh receptors ■ Summary of muscarinic ACh receptor subtypes ■ Therapeutic drugs acting in the PNS ■ Nicotinic receptor agonists ■ Nicotinic receptor antagonists ■ Muscarinic receptor agonists ■ Muscarinic receptor antagonists ■ Effects of anticholinergic drugs on the (mainly) muscarinic actions of ACh

Learning objectives
■ Be able to sketch a simple diagram of the layout of the PNS and label neurotransmitter, site of nicotinic and muscarinic receptors and organ innervated by the PNS.
■ Know the effects of PNS stimulation on the organs innervated.
■ Know the basics of ACh biosynthesis and inactivation, the receptor subtypes and some of the agonists, antagonists and their effects and uses when administered as drugs.
■ Be able to list some anticholinergic drugs and their effects and clinical uses.
■ Know what the anticholinesterases are, and their main autonomic actions and clinical uses.

The parasympathetic division of the ANS
■ Is essential for maintenance of life.
■ Is concerned with proper functioning of the digestive system.
■ Is more localised and limited in each of its various actions than is the sympathetic division.
■ Has efferent nervous outflows from the cranial (midbrain and medulla) and sacral regions of the brain and spinal cord.
■ Usually has relatively long preganglionic fibres that synapse in ganglia close to or on the target organ.
■ Usually has relatively short postganglionic fibres which innervate the target organ.

- Uses ACh as neurotransmitter, released in the ganglia from nerve terminals and acting on nicotinic postsynaptic receptors on the postganglionic nerve fibre.
- Uses ACh as neurotransmitter released from postganglionic nerve terminals and acting on postsynaptic muscarinic receptors on target tissue cells.
- Operates through muscarinic and nicotinic ACh receptors.

Anatomical layout of the PNS

- Cranio-sacral outflows
  - cranial outflow nerves:
    - III, VII (chorda tympani or facial), IX (glossopharyngeal), X (vagus)
  - sacral outflow nerves:
    - sacral outflow nerves, S2, S3, S4.

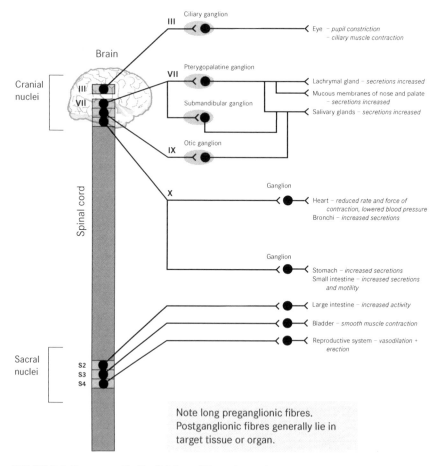

FIGURE 8.1 Parasympathetic division of the autonomic nervous system.

Actions of the PNS on tissues
(*see* Figure 8.1)

Biosynthesis and metabolism of acetylcholine
(*see* Figure 8.2)

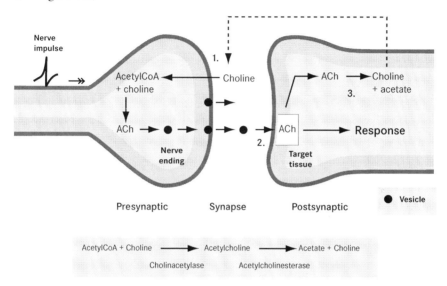

FIGURE 8.2 Formation, action and inactivation of acetylcholine at the synapse.

Receptors for acetylcholine
- Nicotinic ACh receptors occur:
  - in ganglia
  - at the neuromuscular junction (*see* p. 50).
- Muscarinic ACh receptors occur:
  - postsynaptic in ganglia, and
  - at postganglionic, pre- and postsynaptic sites at synapses between the nerve terminal and tissues innervated by the PNS.
- Subtypes of muscarinic receptors identified (at time of writing) are:
  - M1   M2   M3   M4   M5.

Ganglionic muscarinic ACh receptors
- Are present in both sympathetic and parasympathetic ganglia.
- Are located postsynaptically.
- Mediate recovery of the postsynaptic neurone after depolarisation via subtypes M1 (mediates the slow EPSP)* and M2 (mediates the IPSP).

---

* EPSP: excitatory postsynaptic potential; IPSP: inhibitory postsynaptic potential.

Postganglionic muscarinic ACh receptors

- Are present at the postganglionic, presynaptic nerve terminal and postsynaptic on the tissue innervated:
    - presynaptic muscarinic ACh receptors (autoreceptors) regulate ACh release from the nerve terminal
    - postsynaptic muscarinic ACh receptors on the target tissue (e.g. heart muscle cell) mediate the normal response of the tissue to parasympathetic stimulation.

Summary of muscarinic ACh receptor subtypes

MUSCARINIC RECEPTOR	TISSUES	2ND MESSENGER SYSTEM (S)	EFFECT
M1	• CNS • exocrine glands • ganglion (slow EPSP)	• IP3 system activation	• promotes secretions • ganglion recovery • CNS actions
M2	• cardiac muscle	• inhibition of adenylate cyclase–cAMP system	• decreases conduction velocity and heart rate • slows sinoatrial depolarisation
M3	• glandular tissue • smooth muscle of lungs, blood vessels, GIT	• IP3 system activation	• promote secretions • promotes bronchoconstriction and vasodilation • increases GIT motility • dilates sphincters
M4	• CNS	• inhibition of adenylate cyclase–cyclic AMP system	• CNS inhibitory actions
M5	• CNS (at time of writing)	• IP3 system activation	• unknown

Therapeutic drugs acting in the PNS

- In the ganglion
    - ACh nicotinic receptor agonists
    - ACh nicotinic receptor antagonists.
- On the target tissue
    - ACh muscarinic receptor agonists
    - ACh muscarinic receptor antagonists
    - Anticholinesterase drugs that block ACh breakdown.

Nicotinic receptor agonists
- ACh.
- Nicotine.
- Nicotine derivatives (potentially useful for Parkinson's disease, Alzheimer's disease and chronic pain), e.g. epibatidine (extracted from *Epipedobates tricolour*, and Ecuadorian frog) and epiboxidine.

Nicotinic receptor antagonists*
- At the ganglion
  - Hexamethonium.

Muscarinic receptor agonists
- ACh.
- Muscarine.
- Pilocarpine (used to treat glaucoma).

Muscarinic receptor antagonists
- Natural sources
  - atropine (extracted from *Atropa belladonna* (Deadly nightshade))
  - scopolamine (L-hyoscine).
- Synthetic derivatives (not comprehensive)
  - dicyclomine
  - oxybutynin
  - pirenzepine
  - tiotropium
  - tropicamide (short-acting).

Effects of anticholinergic drugs on the (mainly) muscarinic actions of ACh
- Clinical uses of anticholinergic drugs
  - antidote to organophosphorus poisoning
  - antipsychotics
  - antispasmodics in the GIT
  - bronchodilators in asthma
  - treatment of irritable bowel syndrome
  - alleviation of motion sickness
  - dilators of pupils in eye examination (e.g. tropicamide)
  - treatment of diabetic neuropathies
  - treatment of Parkinson's disease
  - premedication for surgery

---

* Note: there are nicotinic receptors at the neuromuscular junction, whose antagonists are dealt with separately (*see* p. 51).

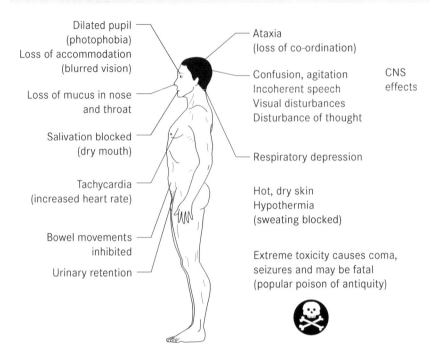

Dilated pupil (photophobia)
Loss of accommodation (blurred vision)

Loss of mucus in nose and throat

Salivation blocked (dry mouth)

Tachycardia (increased heart rate)

Bowel movements inhibited

Urinary retention

Ataxia (loss of co-ordination)

Confusion, agitation
Incoherent speech
Visual disturbances
Disturbance of thought

CNS effects

Respiratory depression

Hot, dry skin
Hypothermia (sweating blocked)

Extreme toxicity causes coma, seizures and may be fatal (popular poison of antiquity)

FIGURE 8.4 Effects of anticholinergic drugs.

- treatment of rhinorrhoea
- treatment of urinary incontinence.
- Anticholinesterase drugs
  - block the enzyme acetylcholinesterase, which breaks down ACh (*see* Figure 8.2)
  - are of two kinds:
    - reversible, e.g. edrophonium
    - irreversible (little or no therapeutic use), e.g. organophosphorus compounds.
  - for clinical use, may be classified as:
    - short-acting, e.g. edrophonium
    - medium-duration action, e.g. physostigmine, neostigmine, pyridostigmine.
  - will block the breakdown of ACh and prolong its actions at:
    - nicotinic ACh receptors in autonomic ganglia
    - muscarinic receptors of the parasympathetic division of the ANS
    - the neuromuscular junction (*see* p. 51 for more details of their actions and uses)
    - ACh receptors in the CNS.

- Autonomic effects of anticholinesterases
  (Effects reflect enhancement of autonomic actions of ACh)
  - cardiovascular actions:
    - bradycardia (slowing of the heart)
    - hypotension.
  - respiratory actions:
    - bronchoconstriction.
  - secretory actions:
    - salivation
    - bronchial secretions increased
    - lacrimation.
  - gastrointestinal tract:
    - increased peristaltic movements
    - increased secretions.
  - the eye:
    - fall in intraocular pressure
    - accommodation for near vision becomes fixed
    - pupillary constriction.
- Clinical uses of antocholinesterases
  - Myasthenia gravis (*see* p. 54).
  - Reversal of muscle relaxant action after general anaesthesia.
  - Treatment of glaucoma (pilocarpine, a muscarinic agonist is usually preferred).
  - Treatment of Alzheimer's disease (e.g. donezepil).

Chapter 8 Quiz

ANSWER T (TRUE) OR F (FALSE)

1. The PNS is not essential for life. ☐
2. PNS efferent outflows are via craniosacral regions. ☐
3. The PNS:
   Is necessary for digestive function. ☐
   Usually has long preganglionic efferent nerve fibres. ☐
   Uses acetylcholine as its major neurotransmitter. ☐
   Operates through nicotinic and muscarinic ACh receptors. ☐
4. PNS stimulation:
   Causes pupillary dilation. ☐
   Causes increased salivation. ☐

Increases heart rate and force of contraction. ☐

Increases bronchial secretions. ☐

Promotes GIT motility. ☐

Inhibits bladder smooth muscle contraction. ☐

Blocks penile vasodilatation and erection. ☐

5. In the PNS, nicotinic ACh receptors occur in the ganglion. ☐

6. In the PNS, muscarinic ACh receptors occur in the ganglion. ☐

7. In the PNS, muscarinic receptors occur on target tissues. ☐

8. Ganglionic muscarinic receptors mediate postsynaptic recovery after depolarisation of the neurone. ☐

9. Postsynaptic ACh receptors regulate ACh release from nerves. ☐

10. M2 ACh muscarinic receptors occur in heart muscle. ☐

11. Nicotinic agonists are used to treat Parkinson's disease. ☐

12. Pilocarpine, a muscarinic antagonist, is used to treat glaucoma. ☐

13. Atropine is a muscarinic antagonist. ☐

14. Tropicamide is a short-acting antimuscarinic drug. ☐

15. Anticholinergic drugs block the actions of atropine. ☐

16. Anticholinergic drugs are used:

As GIT antispasmodics. ☐

For motion sickness. ☐

To dilate the pupil for eye examinations. ☐

As premedication before operations. ☐

To treat polyuria. ☐

17. Anticholinesterase drugs block the action of acetylcholine. ☐

18. Anticholinesterase drugs:

Cause slowing of the heart (bradycardia). ☐

Hypotension. ☐

Bronchoconstriction. ☐

Decreased peristalsis. ☐

Fall in intraocular pressure. ☐

19. Clinical uses of anticholinesterases include:

Treatment of myasthenia gravis. ☐

Postoperative reversal of muscle relaxant action. ☐

Occasionally treatment of glaucoma. ☐

Treatment of Alzheimer's disease. ☐

The autonomic system III: sympathetic division (SNS)

Learning objectives ■ The sympathetic division of the ANS ■ Anatomical layout of the SNS ■ Actions of the SNS on tissues and organs ■ Adrenoceptor classification ■ Current knowledge of α_1-adrenoceptor subtype function ■ Current knowledge of α_2-adrenoceptor subtype function ■ Release, action and inactivation of norepinephrine ■ Biosynthesis of norepinephrine and epinephrine ■ Metabolism of epinephrine and norepinephrine (NE) ■ Therapeutic drugs acting through the SNS

Learning objectives

■ Be able to sketch the layout of the SNS.
■ Know the main points about SNS actions on the different systems.
■ Have knowledge of the main classification subdivisions of the adrenoceptors.
■ Be able to sketch the events at the adrenergic synapse following arrival of the nerve impulse.
■ Know the pathways of synthesis and inactivation of NE and epinephrine.
■ Be able to give at least one example of a therapeutic drug and its adrenoceptor site.

The sympathetic division of the ANS

■ Is not essential for maintenance of life.
■ Is concerned with initiation of the 'fight or flight reflex'.
■ Is *less* localised and *less* limited in each of its various actions than is the parasympathetic division.
■ Has efferent nervous outflows from the thoraco-lumbar regions of the spinal cord.
■ Usually has *short* preganglionic fibres that synapse in ganglia close to the spinal cord.
■ Usually has relatively *long* postganglionic fibres which innervate the target organ.
■ Like the parasympathetic division, uses ACh as neurotransmitter, which is released in the ganglia from nerve terminals and acts on nicotinic postsynaptic receptors on the postganglionic nerve fibre.

- Unlike the parasympathetic division, uses norepinephrine as neuro-transmitter which is released from postganglionic nerve terminals and acts on postsynaptic α- and β-adrenoceptors receptors on target tissue cells.

Anatomical layout of the SNS

- Origin of sympathetic nerves: intermediolateral cell column of the vertebral column.
- Spinal cord segments of origin: thoraco-lumbar region of the cord from T1–L2, 3.

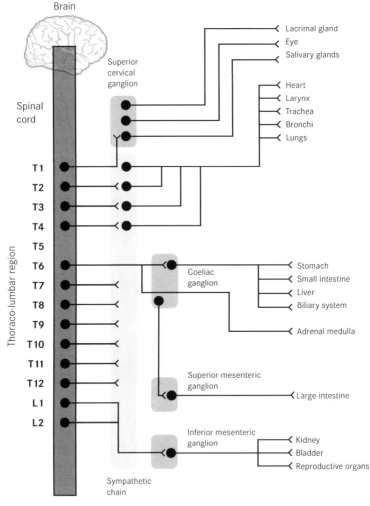

FIGURE 9.1 Sympathetic division of the autonomic nervous system (one side only is shown).

Actions of the SNS on tissues and organs

- Cardiovascular system
  - heart: increases rate and force of cardiac muscle contraction through β_1 receptors
  - blood vessels: vasoconstriction in (e.g.) skin via α_1-adrenoceptors; vasodilatation in arterioles supplying (e.g.) skeletal muscle via β_2-adrencoeptors.
- Skeletal muscle
  - glycogenolysis via β_2-adrenoceptors
  - tremor via β_3-adrenoceptors, thermogenesis
  - enhanced speed and force of contraction via β_2-adrenoceptors.
- Bronchi
  - dilation of bronchial tree via β_2-adrenoceptors.
- Fat
  - lipolysis via β_3-adrenoceptors, thermogenesis.
- Liver
  - glycogenolysis via β_2-adrenoceptors.
- Pancreas
  - insulin secretion.
- Bladder
  - urination reflex via α_1-adrenoceptors
  - smooth muscle constriction in bladder neck via α_1-adrenoceptors.
- Pupil
  - dilation of the pupil by contraction of the radial muscles via α_1-adrenoceptors.
- Reproductive system
  - female
    - non-pregnant uterine smooth muscle *relaxation* via β_2-adrenoceptors
    - pregnant uterine smooth muscle *contraction* via α_1-adrenoceptors.
  - male
    - ejaculation via α_1-adrenoceptors
    - contraction of prostate via α_1-adrenoceptors in fibromuscular stroma and capsule of the prostate gland.

Adrenoceptor classification

- Alpha-adrenoceptors: α1A, α1B, α1D, α2A, α2B, α2C.
- Beta-adrenoceptors: β1, β2, β3.

Current knowledge of α_1-adrenoceptor subtype function[*]

- α_{1A}

---

[*] Studies are from different species, which further complicates matters.

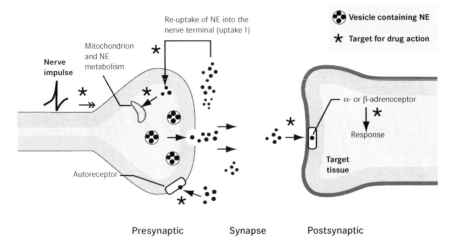

FIGURE 9.2 Release, action and inactivation of norepinephrine (NE) at the synapse.

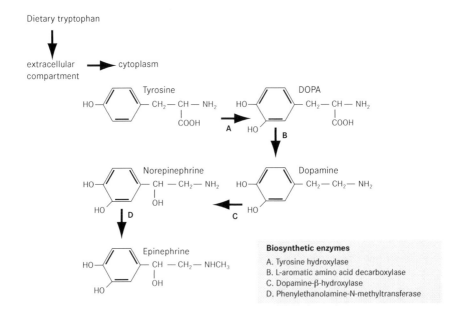

FIGURE 9.3 Synthesis of norepinephrine and epinephrine.

- mediation of cardiac hypertrophy
- mediation of positive ionotropic actions
- mediation of metabolic effects
- mediation of vasoconstriction.
- α_{1B}
  - mediation of intracellular mobilisation of Ca^{2+}.
- α_{1D}*
  - mediation of vasoconstriction.

Current knowledge of α_2-adrenoceptor subtype function

- α_{2A}
  - meditation of effects in the spinal cord
  - mediation of central antihypertensive actions of α_2-adrenoceptor agonist drugs, e.g. clonidine.

Release, action and inactivation of norepinephrine

1. Action potential (AP) arrives at nerve terminal and causes fusion of vesicle with cell membrane and NE is released into synaptic cleft.
2. Neurotransmitter diffuses to:
   (a) postsynaptic adrenoceptors and activates response
   (b) presynaptic membrane where it:
     - is actively taken back up into the nerve terminal (uptake 1) and metabolised in the mitochondrion
     - is taken up into the postsynaptic neurone (uptake 2)
     - binds to presynaptic NE autoreceptors which limit further release of NE.
3. NE is metabolised to inactive metabolites by the mitochondrial enzyme monoamine oxidase and by the cytoplasmic enzyme catechol-O-methyltransferase (*see* also below).

Biosynthesis of norepinephrine and epinephrine

- Tyrosine hydroxylase catalyses tyrosine =>DOPA
  - rate-limiting step inhibited by NE
  - enzyme found only in catecholamine-synthesising cells.
- DOPA decarboxylase catalyses DOPA => dopamine
  - enzyme more widespread; catalyses decarboxylation of L-aromatic amino acids
  - is a target for drugs to treat Parkinson's disease (*see* below).
- Dopamine β-hydroxylase catalyses dopamine => norepinephrine (NE)
  - occurs in synaptic vesicles

---

* Now designated $\alpha1_{A/D}$

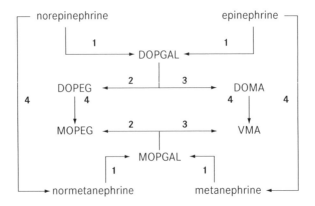

DOPGAL: 3,4-dihydroxyphenylglycoaldehyde
DOPEG: 3,4-dihydroxyphenlyethyleneglycol
DOMA: 3,4-dihydroxymandelic acid
MOPGAL: 3-methoxy-4-hydroxyphenylglycoaldehyde
MOPEG: 3-methoxy-4-hydroxyphenylethyleneglycol
VMA: 3-methox-4-hydroxymandelic acid

1: Monoamine oxidase (MAO)
2: Aldehyde reductase
3: Aldehyde dehydrogenase
4: Catechol-O-methyltrasferase (COMT)

FIGURE 9.4 Metabolism of the catecholamines.

- membrane-bound enzyme
- inhibited by disulfiram (Antabuse), a drug used to treat alcoholism.*
- Phenylethanolamine-N-methyltransferase catalyses Ne => epinephrine
  - enzyme occurs in the adrenal medullary cells which produce epinephrine
  - occurs also in brain.

Metabolism of epinephrine and norepinephrine (NE)

- Monoamine oxidase (MAO)
  - occurs bound to the outer membrane of mitochondria
  - converts NE and epinephrine to an inactive aldehyde (DOPGAL)

---

* Disulfiram is used to discourage alcoholics; it blocks acetaldehyde dehydrogenase, which converts acetaldehyde, an alcohol metabolite, to acetic acid. Acetaldehyde build-up gives acute discomfort, to put it mildly, and further alcohol consumption becomes less likely.

- exists in 2 isoforms in neurones: MAO-A and MAO-B
- MAO-A also occurs in GIT, liver and placenta
- MAO-B also breaks down dopamine.*
- Catechol-O-methyltransferase (COMT)
  - acts on NE, epinephrine and dopamine
  - is a target for drug action, e.g. entacapone is used in Parkinson's disease together with dopa decarboxylase inhibitors carbidopa and benserazide to protect L-Dopa (*see* p. 207).

THERAPEUTIC DRUGS ACTING THROUGH THE SNS
(For information on ganglion-active drugs *see* p. 34)

DRUGS ACTING THROUGH ALPHA-ADRENOCEPTORS
α_1-adrenoceptor agonists
- Epinephrine.
- Norepinephrine.
- Phenylephrine.
- Xylometazoline.
- Methoxamine.
- Oxymetazoline.
- Tetrahydralazine.

Uses of α_1-adrenoceptor agonists
- Pressor agents (increase blood pressure) to treat shock and hypotension, e.g. phenylephrine.
- Nasal decongestants (cause nasal vasoconstriction), e.g. xylometazoline, oxymetazoline, phenylephrine.

Adverse effects of α_1-adrenoceptor agonists
- Reflex bradycardia (slowing of the heart).
- Systemic vasoconstriction, thus increasing the heart's workload, which can cause pain for angina sufferers.
- Headaches.
- Central effects, e.g. irritability, restlessness and excitement.
- As nasal decongestants, they can cause rebound vasodilation and nasal congestion on withdrawal (rhinitis medicamentosa); phenylephrine is the safest of the three in this respect.

α_2-adrenoceptor agonists
- Clonidine.
- α-methyldopa.
- Epinephrine.
- Norepinephrine.

---

* This is NB for patients with Parkinson's disease (*see* p. 206) since the MAOI selegiline is specific for MAO-B.

Uses of synthetic α_2-adrenoceptor agonists

- Hypertension, through a central action.
- Menopausal flushing.
- Migraine.
- Tourette's syndrome.[*]

Adverse effects of α_2-adrenoceptor agonists (not comprehensive)

- Bradycardia.
- Depression.
- Euphoria.
- Occasionally impotence.
- Sedation.
- Constipation.
- Dry mouth.
- Fluid retention.
- Raynaud's syndrome.[†]
- Rebound hypertension on abrupt cessation of the drug.

α-adrenoceptor antagonists

- α_1-adrenoceptor antagonists.
- α^2-adrenoceptor antagonists.
- Non-selective α-adrenoceptor antagonists.

α_1-adrenoceptor antagonists[‡]

- Alfuzocin.
- Doxazosin (longer-acting than prazocin).
- Indoramin.
- Prazocin (relatively short-acting; has approximately 1000-fold higher affinity for α_1 than for α_2).
- Tamsulosin.
- Terazocin.

Uses of α_1-adrenoceptor antagonists

- Benign prostatic hyperplasia (e.g. alfuzocin, doxazosin, terazocin).
- Hypertension, usually with other antihypertensive drugs.

Adverse effects of α_1-adrenoceptor antagonists[§]

- Sharp, rapid fall in blood pressure after first dose causing fainting (first dose effect).
- Postural hypotension.
- Vertigo (dizziness and loss of balance).

---

[*] Tourette's syndrome: named after Dr George Gilles de la Tourette; a chronic condition of involuntary movements.
[†] Raynaud's syndrome: icy coldness of extremities, for example fingers and toes, due to vasoconstriction of peripheral arterioles.
[‡] α_1-blockers do also block α_2-adrenoceptors to variable extents; this list is not exhaustive.
[§] Not comprehensive; see British National Formulary (BNF) for more details.

- Nausea and possible vomiting.
- Rhinitis.
- Thrombocytopaenia (platelet reduction in blood).

α_2-adrenoceptor antagonists
- Yohimbine, a plant alkaloid.

DRUGS ACTING THROUGH BETA-ADRENOCEPTORS
Beta agonists
- Mixed β_1 and β_2-adrenoceptors.
- β_1-adrenoceptors.
- β_2-adrenoceptors.

Mixed β_1-and β_2-adrenoceptor agonists[*]
- Epinephrine.
- Norepinephrine.
- Isoprenaline.

β_2-adrenoceptor agonists
- Short-acting.
- Longer-acting.
- Used for treatment of asthma.

Short-acting β_2-adrenoceptor agonists
- Salbutamol.
- Terbutaline.
- Fenoterol (used for reversible airways obstruction).

Longer-acting β_2-adrenoceptor agonists
- Bambuterol.
- Formoterol.
- Salmeterol.

Beta antagonists[†]
- Mixed β_1 and β_2 antagonists:[‡]
  - propranolol
  - nadolol
  - pindolol.
  - carvedilol
  - labetolol

---

[*] Not comprehensive.
[†] Not comprehensive; selective emphasis on currently used β-blockers in the UK.
[‡] More dangerous in asthmatics due to danger of bronchoconstriction through blocking of bronchiolar β_2-adrenoceptors.

- β_1-selective antagonists:
  - acebutolol
  - atenolol
  - bisoprolol
  - celiprolol
  - esmolol
  - metoprolol.
- Drugs acting through blockade of Uptake 1:
  - amphetamines
  - tricyclic antidepressants (*see* pp. 65, 218, 220).

Chapter 9 Quiz

ANSWER T (TRUE) OR F (FALSE)

1. The SNS is not essential for life. ☐
2. SNS efferent outflows are via the thoraco-lumbar cord segments. ☐
3. The SNS:
   Is necessary for the flight or fight reflex. ☐
   Usually has a short preganglionic efferent nerve fibre. ☐
   Uses norepinephrine as its major neurotransmitter. ☐
   Is highly selective in its physiological responses. ☐
4. SNS stimulation:
   Causes pupillary dilation through α_1-adrenoceptors. ☐
   Increases cardiac rate and force of contraction via β_1-adrenoceptors. ☐
   Causes bronchial constriction via β_2-adrenoceptors. ☐
   Causes thermogenesis through lipolysis via β_3-adrenoceptors. ☐
   Constricts the bladder neck to inhibit urination. ☐
   Promotes non-pregnant uterine contractions. ☐
   Enables ejaculation via α_1-adrenoceptors. ☐
5. In the SNS, nicotinic ACh receptors occur in the ganglion. ☐
6. In the SNS, muscarinic ACh receptors occur in the ganglion. ☐
7. In the SNS, muscarinic receptors occur on target tissues. ☐
8. Ganglionic muscarinic receptors mediate postsynaptic recovery after depolarisation of the neurone. ☐
9. Presynaptic α_2-adrenoceptors inhibit NE release from nerves. ☐
10. NE causes glycogenolysis in skeletal muscle via β_2-adrenoceptors. ☐
11. NE action is terminated by Uptake 1 into presynaptic nerves. ☐
12. Uptake 1 is enhanced by amphetamines. ☐
13. Oxymetazoline, used to relieve nasal congestion is an α_1-agonist. ☐
14. NE and epinephrine are metabolised by MAO. ☐
15. NE and epinephrine are also metabolised by COMT. ☐

10 The neuromuscular junction (NMJ)

Learning objectives ■ The neuromuscular junction ■ Structure and function of the neuromuscular junction ■ Functional structure of the nicotinic ACh receptor at the NMJ ■ Drugs that modify neuromuscular transmission ■ Neuromuscular blocking drugs ■ Non-depolarising neuromuscular blocking drugs ■ Depolarising neuromuscular blocking drugs ■ Anticholinesterases

Learning objectives
- Be able to sketch a diagram of the NMJ, showing the key components.
- Know the key events as given here from arrival of the impulse at the terminal to the muscle contraction.
- Be ready to give examples of non-depolarising and depolarising neuromuscular drugs together with examples.
- Be able to explain the main distinction between the terms 'competitive' and 'non-competitive' neuromuscular block.
- Know some of the main precautions and adverse effects of neuromuscular blocking drugs.
- Be able give examples of the various anticholinesterases and to explain briefly how they work.
- Know what anticholinesterases are used for.
- Be able to give examples of irreversible anticholinesterases, the antidote and be aware of the implications of irreversible anticholinesterase action.

The neuromuscular junction
- Is where the efferent motor nerve synapses with muscle, here meaning skeletal muscle.
- Is where the motor nerve impulse is transduced into a postsynaptic action potential which is transduced by the muscle fibre into a muscle contraction.
- Includes:
  - the presynaptic motor nerve terminal
  - the synaptic cleft
  - the motor end plate, the postsynaptic region of the muscle cell membrane.

- Is a target for drugs which:
  - block neuromuscular transmission, thereby causing muscle relaxation
  - enhance neurotransmission, thereby improving skeletal muscle performance.

Structure and function of the neuromuscular junction

1. There is a presynaptic cholinergic nerve terminal, which stores acetylcholine (ACh) as neurotransmitter in vesicles and on arrival of the nerve impulse
2. Takes in Ca^{2+} ions from the cytoplasm, which triggers release of ACh into
3. The synaptic cleft, which is about 2–3 nm wide, across which ACh diffuses to
4. The postsynaptic nicotinic ACh receptor to which ACh binds and triggers
5. An opening of ion channels, allowing Na^+ influx and K^+ efflux at the muscle endplate, which creates
6. An electrochemical gradient across the plasma membrane of the endplate and a
7. Local endplate potential (EPP), which spreads over the entire surface of the muscle fibre, and this triggers a generalised release of Ca^{2+} from the muscle's sarcoplasmic reticulum, thereby triggering
8. Muscle contraction.

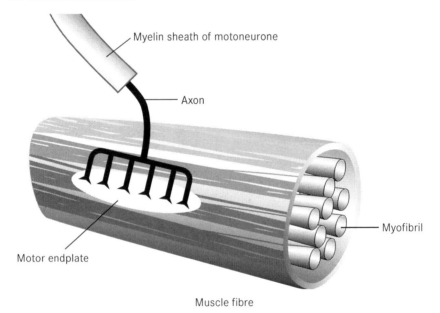

FIGURE 10.1 The motor endplate.

Functional structure of the nicotinic ACh receptor at the NMJ

- Polymeric, transmembrane receptor consisting of five subunits, including two α-subunits, each binding a molecule of ACh.
- Binding opens an ion channel in the receptor allowing Na^+ to flow into the cell.

Drugs that modify neuromuscular transmission

- Neuromuscular blocking drugs – block neuromuscular transmission.
- Anticholinesterase drugs – enhance neuromuscular transmission.

Neuromuscular blocking drugs

- Non-depolarising neuromuscular blocking drugs.
- Depolarising blocking drugs.
- Used mainly to relax skeletal muscle during surgical operations.

Non-depolarising neuromuscular blocking drugs

- Include tubocurarine, the alkaloid extracted from curare.
- Are competitive antagonists of acetylcholine at postsynaptic ACh receptor sites, i.e. increasing the concentration of ACh will displace the blocker and *vice versa.*
- Are usually reversibly bound, i.e. will dissociate from the receptor.
- May also bind to presynaptic ACh receptors.
- May bind to either one or both α-subunits of the ACh receptor.
- Start to block neuromuscular action when ~ 75% of ACh receptors are occupied by antagonist.
- Produce a complete block when > 90% of ACh receptors are occupied by antagonist.
- Are not metabolised at the NMJ, and duration of block depends on systemic clearance time.
- Have no sedative or analgesic actions.
- Have low potential for malignant hyperthermia.
- Usually have low allergic potential.
- Effects are reduced by treatment with anticholinesterases (*see* below).

Classes of non-depolarising blocking drugs

- Aminosteroids.
- Benzylisoquinolines.

Aminosteroids

DRUG	ONSET	DURATION
rocuronium	± 2 minutes	± 35 minutes
pancuronium	± 4 minutes	± 50 minutes
vecuronium	± 3 minutes	± 25 minutes

Precautions*

* Allergic cross-reactivity between different muscle relaxants.
* Activity prolonged in patients with myasthenia gravis.
* Use with caution in pregnancy.

Adverse effects

* Hypertension and tachycardia (pancuronium and rocuronium at high doses; sympathomimetic and vagolytic† actions).
* Little histamine-releasing effect.

Benzylisoquinolines

DRUG	ONSET	DURATION
tubocurarine	± 3-5 minutes	± 30-60 minutes
atracurium	± 2-4 minutes	± 25-35 minutes
cisatracurium	± 2-4 minutes	± 25-45 minutes
mivacurium	2-4 minutes	10-25 minutes
gallamine	1-2 minutes	15-30 minutes

Precautions

* With obese patients, doses should be calculated for ideal body weight and not actual weight due to dangers of overdose.
* Causes histamine release due partly to products of enzymatic breakdown by plasma cholinesterase.
* Activity is prolonged in patients with myasthenia gravis.
* Patients with low plasma cholinesterase should be titrated‡ for dose.
* Gallamine is vagolytic and sympathomimetic and should not be used in patients with renal disease or impairment.
* Use with caution in pregnancy.

Safety note: Check for crystallisation of drug in the syringe as injection can cause tissue damage.

---

* Not comprehensive.
† Vagolytic: inhibition of the vagus (10th cranial) nerve.
‡ Titrated: here means the determination of a safe, low dose for that patient.

Adverse effects

* Hypotension and bradycardia (heart slowing) due to histamine release.
* Increased possibility of histamine release and hypotension with higher doses of mivacurium (>1.5 mg/Kg).

Depolarising neuromuscular blocking drugs

* Suxamethonium (also called succinylcholine)
  * chemical nature and action:
    * consists of two molecules of ACh linked together
    * due to similarity to ACh, binds ACh receptor and causes depolarisation, resulting in fine tremor or 'fasciculation' followed by flaccid paralysis due to prolonged depolarisation through slow dissociation from the receptor
    * the only drug of this class clinically used.
  * indications for use:
    * rapid onset of neuromuscular block needed, e.g. in emergency incubation of the trachea
    * short duration of action needed, e.g. when fast recovery of neuromuscular function is required.
  * administration:
    * should be administered *after* induction of anaesthesia because fasciculation may be very painful
    * IV administration causes fast paralysis (onset often < 1minute); duration 2-6 minutes
    * IM administration causes slower onset; used when IV not possible, e.g. babies
    * IV infusion administration after initial IV dose for prolonged neuromuscular block.
  * precautions:
    * pregnancy
    * neuromuscular or respiratory disease
    * raised intra-ocular pressure
    * avoid in patients with penetrating eye injury due to the risk of expulsion of the vitreous contents
    * severe sepsis which may result in hyperkalaemia (raised blood potassium; suxamethonium can produce hyperkalaemia).
  * contraindications:
    * patients with inefficient plasma cholinesterase activity, usually due to genetically abnormal cholinesterase enzyme structure

- ◆ patients with family history of malignant hyperthermia[*]
- ◆ severe liver disease, resulting in decreased production of plasma cholinesterase
- ◆ hyperkalaemia, because suxamethonium increases plasma K^+ and hyperkalaemia can precipitate arrhythmias; susceptible patients include those with severe burns, especially if used after the first 2–3 hours of burn occurrence; patients with muscular dystrophy and paraplegic patients; patients with severe sepsis.
- ▌ adverse effects of suxamethonium:
  - ◆ cardiovascular problems: cardiac arrest, tachycardia, arrhythmias, hypotension or hypertension
  - ◆ anaphylactic reactions
  - ◆ increased gastric pressure
  - ◆ post-operative muscle pain
  - ◆ respiratory depression
  - ◆ hyperkalaemia
  - ◆ myoglobinaemia
  - ◆ myoglobinurea
  - ◆ flushes
  - ◆ skin rashes.

Note: unlike the case for non-depolarising neuromuscular blocking drugs, whose effects are reversed by anticholinesterases, the actions of depolarising neuromuscular blocking drugs, e.g. suxamethonium, are actually enhanced by anticholinesterases.

Anticholinesterases

- ▒ Inhibit the breakdown of ACh by the enzyme acetylcholinesterase (AChE).
- ▒ Prolong and enhance the action of ACh at its receptor and of its effects on the tissues, e.g. the neuromuscular junction, the ganglia and on tissues innervated by the PNS or SNS (e.g. sweat glands) which receive cholinergic innervation.
- ▒ Are used to treat conditions such as myasthenia gravis.
- ▒ Are used to treat Alzheimer's disease.
- ▒ Have been used in warfare as nerve gases and are used in insecticides.
- ▒ Have been classified into various classes:
  - ▌ reversible (therapeutic use)
  - ▌ irreversible (no therapeutic use, e.g. insecticides, nerve gases).

---

[*] Malignant hyperthermia: rapid onset of very high fever with muscle rigidity during administration of general anaesthesia, in genetically susceptible patients; suxamethonium and the general anaesthetic halothane are especially likely to precipitate malignant hyperthermia.

Reversible anticholinesterases

- Short-acting:
  - edrophonium.
- Medium-long acting:
  - donezepil
  - physostigmine
  - pyridostigmine
  - galantamine
  - neostigmine*
  - rivastigmine.

Therapeutic uses of reversible anticholinesterases

- Diagnostic of myasthenia gravis[†] with short-acting edrophonium, which produces a transient improvement and a rapid relapse.[‡]
- Treatment of myasthenia gravis with medium-longer-acting reversible anticholinesterases, e.g. pyridostigmine (~ 3-6 hours duration).
- Treatment of Alzheimer's disease with the medium-duration, reversible anticholinesterases, e.g. donezepil, rivastigmine, which cross the blood–brain barrier.
- Post-operative reactivation of GIT and bladder muscles following surgery, e.g. neostigmine.
- Treatment of open-angle glaucoma with short-acting physostigmine, together with pilocarpine, a muscarinic agonist (β-blockers and prostaglandins are also used topically).

Note: *See* the BNF[§] for precautions and adverse effects for these agents.

Irreversible anticholinesterases

- Have virtually no therapeutic use.
- Combine irreversibly with ACh and new enzyme has to be synthesised.
- Produce symptoms representative of nicotinic, muscarinic and CNS over-activity.
- Can possibly be reversed if patient is treated with pralidoxime within about 6 hours of poisoning and higher doses may be tried if longer times have elapsed; atropine, diazepam and artificial respiration are often also necessary.
- Are used as insecticides, e.g. malathion, parathion.
- Have been used in warfare, e.g. Sarin.

---

[*] Drugs such as neostigmine are actually competitive substrates for AChE.
[†] Autoimmune disease when ACh receptors are attacked by the immune system, resulting in muscle weakness and exhaustion.
[‡] A useful test to distinguish between myasthenia gravis (MG) and anticholinesterase poisoning, for example with irreversible anticholinesterase insecticides. Patient with MG has transient improvement but poisoned patient shows no improvement.
[§] BNF: British National Formulary.

Chapter 10 Quiz

ANSWER T (TRUE) OR F (FALSE)

1. The motor endplate is postsynaptic on the muscle membrane. ☐
2. The motor endplate is a target for neuromuscular blockers. ☐
3. The main events at the NMJ resulting in ACh release are:
    Arrival of the impulse at the motor nerve terminal, which ☐
    Triggers Ca^{2+} influx into the cytoplasm, which ☐
    Triggers fusion of vesicles with nerve cell membrane and ☐
    Release of epinephrine into the synaptic cleft. ☐
4. The main NMJ postsynaptic events are:
    Binding of ACh to ACh receptors on the motor endplate, which ☐
    Causes ion channel opening and Na^+ influx, which ☐
    Causes a transmembrane electrochemical gradient and ☐
    Generation of a local endplate potential, which ☐
    Spreads over the muscle fibre and triggers ☐
    A generalised release of intracellular Na^+ ions ☐
    Resulting in muscle contraction. ☐
5. The nicotinic NMJ ACh receptor has 2 ACh-binding α subunits. ☐
6. Non-depolarising NMJ blocking drugs:
    Include aminosteroids and benzylisoquinolines. ☐
    Are usually irreversibly bound to the ACh receptor. ☐
    Are competitive antagonists of ACh at the ACh receptor. ☐
    May bind also to presynaptic ACh receptors. ☐
    Action duration depends mainly on systemic clearance. ☐
    Have low potential for reactive hyperthermia. ☐
    Action is reversed by increasing local ACh concentrations. ☐
    Include pancuronium, rocuronium and vecuronium. ☐
7. Aminosteroids have high HIS* release potential. ☐
8. They can cause sympathomimetic and vagolytic effects. ☐
9. These include tachycardia and hypertension. ☐
10. They have powerful analgesic or sedative action. ☐
11. Benzylisoquinoline NMJ blocking drugs:
    Include atracurium, cisatracurium, gallamine, mivacurium. ☐
    Can cause histamine release with bradycardia and hypotension. ☐
    Action is prolonged in patients with myasthenia gravis. ☐

Require dose titration with low plasma cholinesterase patients. ☐

Should be used with caution, if at all, in pregnant patients. ☐

12. Suxamethonium:

Is the only depolarising NMJ blocker used now.[†] ☐

Consists of three molecules of ACh joined together. ☐

On binding to the ACh receptor causes initial tremor before block. ☐

Is used when fast NMJ block is needed, e.g. emergency use. ☐

Is used when fast recovery from block is required. ☐

Should be administered after induction.[‡] ☐

Should be avoided with penetrating eye injury. ☐

Is contraindicated with recent burn injuries. ☐

Can cause arrhythmias and cardiac arrest. ☐

13. Anticholinesterase drugs:

Enhance the breakdown of ACh by acetylcholinesterase. ☐

May be reversible or irreversible. ☐

Are used to treat myasthenia gravis by prolonging NMJ ACh action. ☐

Are used to treat Alzheimer's disease. ☐

14. Reversible anticholinesterases may be:

Short-acting, e.g. neostigmine. ☐

Of medium duration, e.g. rivastigmine. ☐

Used to diagnose and treat myasthenia gravis. ☐

Used to treat open-angle glaucoma. ☐

Used to re-activate the GIT after surgery. ☐

* HIS: histamine.
† At the time of writing.
‡ Tremors or fasciculation caused by suxamethonium before block can be painful.

11 Myasthenia

Learning objectives
- Know what the term myasthenia means.
- Be able to list the different forms of myasthenia gravis (MG).
- Know something of the symptoms, causes, diagnosis and treatment of MG.
- Be aware of the different types of juvenile MG.
- Know what is meant by the Lambert-Eaton myasthenic syndrome and of its link to cancer.

A definition of myasthenia
Debilitating weakness and fatigue of voluntary muscle.

Forms of myasthenia
- Myasthenia gravis.
- Neonatal myasthenia gravis.
- Lambert-Eaton myasthenia gravis.
- Juvenile myasthenia gravis.
- Congenital myasthenia gravis.

Myasthenia gravis summary
- Chronic illness.
- No cure at time of writing.
- Symptoms include:
  - initially, intermittent ptosis (drooping eyelids), diplopia (double vision), dysarthria (difficulty speaking), dysphagia (difficulty swallowing), neck muscle weakness (head falls back or forward)
  - generalised, spreading muscle weakness with 12 months of onset in legs, arms (usually worst affected) and trunk
  - progressive severity as day progresses
  - myasthenia crisis
    - an emergency generated by failure of respiratory muscle, or choking due to aspiration of food and pneumonia
    - caused by (e.g.) surgery, abrupt cessation of corticosteroids (*see* below), viral infection, intense physical activity, emotional stress

♦ with danger of asphyxiation due to choking after food aspiration, respiratory failure due to respiratory muscle failure.

▦ Cause is autoimmune attack at the NMJ resulting in failure of the nerve impulse to generate an effective postsynaptic response.

▦ Causative agents identified are:
- antibodies to the nicotinic ACh receptor at the NMJ
- antibodies to a muscle-specific tyrosine kinase (MuSK) which mediates AChR clustering*
- antibodies to other proteins which mediate normal NMJ transmission.

▦ Diagnosis includes:
- detection of circulating antibodies to AChR or MuSK
- detection of antibodies to other proteins, e.g. actin
- electrodiagnostic tests of NMJ function
- edrophonium, a short-acting anticholinesterase, which causes transient improvement.

▦ Treatment aims at restoration of normal movement as far as possible, using:
- anticholinesterases, e.g. distigmine, neostigmine or pyridostigmine, to increase ACh concentrations at the motor endplate
- immunosuppressants, e.g. corticosteroids such as prednisolone alone or together with non-steroidal immunosuppressants, e.g. azathioprine, to reduce prednisolone dose; other immunosuppressants used include cyclophosphamide and cyclosporin
- plasmapheresis, which is drawing of blood from the patient and removal of the plasma and transfusing the blood cells back into the patient; this reduces damaging antibodies in the circulation
- EN101, an antisense oligonucleotide which interferes with the expression of a form of AChE that enhances the breakdown of ACh at the synapse – still in a developmental stage
- thymectomy, a surgical intervention of uncertain value; the thymus is a source of immune-active T-cells.

Note: Many patients will need combined corticosteroid and azathioprine therapy.

Juvenile myasthenia gravis

▦ Appears before 20 years of age, there are three main types:
- congenital MG: presents within first postnatal year and lifelong; autosomal recessive;† rare, no autoimmune involvement

---

* AChR clustering is the normal developmental concentration of ACh receptors at the motor endplate.
† Autosomal: involves any chromosome other than a sex chromosome. Recessive: a gene representing a trait not expressed unless present on two chromosomes, one from each parent.

- transient neonatal MG: may present very temporarily in infants born to mothers with MG; no later occurrence in offspring ever reported
- juvenile MG: comprises ~ 10% of MG; restricted mainly to adolescent Caucasian girls; lifelong with intermittent remission.

■ Symptoms that may occur:
- fatigue, poor suck in babies, respiratory difficulties, dysphagia, poor vision, ptosis (prognosis in juvenile MG generally good with disappearance of symptoms with time).

■ Diagnosis:
- edrophonium test
- electromyography (EMG)* and single fibre EMG
- serology, but not always helpful as antibodies are not usually expressed in prepubertal MG.

■ Treatment options:
- anticholinesterases
- thymectomy (more effective than in adults, with no reliable reports of later adverse consequences)
- azathioprine sometimes used (corticosteroids not advisable, especially due to growth-stunting effects).

Note: Plasmapheresis is a problem in children and infants due to their small blood volumes.

Lambert-Eaton myasthenic syndrome
■ Is a relatively rare disorder of transmission at the NMJ.
■ Is caused by autoimmune attack on presynaptic voltage-gated Ca^{2+} channels.
■ Results from failure of or reduced ACh release from the nerve terminal.
■ Is characterised by progressive muscle weakness, commonly trunk and leg, and less commonly bulbar,[†] ptosis and respiratory system; reduced or lost reflexes.
■ Often precedes small cell lung carcinoma; may involve other cancers.
■ Is treated with:
- immunosuppressants
- plasmapheresis
- high dose IV immunoglobulin
- drugs that promote ACh release and action, e.g. pyridostigmine, an anticholinesterase, or diaminopyridine.
■ Usually signals a malignancy.

---

* EMG: continuous electrical recording from electrodes inserted into muscle.
† Bulbar: here refers to the conjunctiva; generally refers to rounded or bulbar structures.

Note: 3,4-diaminopyridine increases ACh release from nerve terminals and blocks potassium conductance, thereby prolonging the action potential at the nerve terminal, and causing increased ACh release. Adverse effects include fatigue, headache, insomnia and it can cause seizures. It is contraindicated in epilepsy and at time of writing is still undergoing tests in the UK.

Chapter 11 Quiz

ANSWER T (TRUE) OR F (FALSE)

1. Myasthenia gravis (MG) is a debilitating disease of smooth muscle. ☐
2. MG is an autoimmune disease that targets the NMJ.* ☐
3. Important targets for antibody production include:
   The acetylcholine receptor at the NMJ. ☐
   Nerve-specific tyrosine kinase (MuSK). ☐
4. Symptoms of myasthenia gravis include:
   Drooping eyelids (ptosis). ☐
   Double vision (diplopia). ☐
   Speech difficulties (dysarthria). ☐
   Difficulty swallowing (dysphagia). ☐
   Generalised muscle weakness. ☐
   Respiratory distress. ☐
5. Antibodies block ACh binding to its receptor at the NMJ. ☐
6. Diagnostic procedures include:
   Detection of circulating antibodies to the ACh receptor. ☐
   ECG. ☐
   Detection of circulating antibodies to MuSK.† ☐
7. Treatment of myasthenia gravis employs:
   Anticholinesterases displace antibodies from ACh receptors. ☐
   Immunosuppressants, e.g. corticosteroids. ☐
   Plasmapheresis. ☐
   Thymectomy. ☐
8. Juvenile myasthenia gravis may be diagnosed using edrophonium. ☐
9. Juvenile MG has similar treatment strategies as for adults. ☐
10. Lambert-Eaton myasthenic syndrome (LEMS) involves lack of ACh. ☐
11. LEMS requires drugs that potentiate ACh release and action. ☐

* NMJ: neuromuscular junction.
† MuSK: muscle-specific tyrosine kinase.

12 5-hydroxytryptamine (5-HT; serotonin)

Learning objectives ■ 5-hydroxytryptamine (5-HT; serotonin) ■ Biosynthesis of 5-HT ■ Currently perceived significance of 5-HT ■ Clinical significance of 5-HT ■ Release of 5-HT from neurones ■ Termination of action of 5-HT ■ Metabolism of 5-HT ■ 5-HT receptors ■ 5-HT as a neurotransmitter and neuromodulator in the gastrointestinal tract (GIT)

Learning objectives

■ Be able to give an account of the occurrence, biosynthesis, release and metabolism of 5-HT.
■ Know the given features of 5-HT release and termination of action of 5-HT at the synapse and the clinical significance for drug action.
■ Read through the formidable and growing list of 5-HT receptor subtypes.
■ Be able to give an account of the occurrence and role of 5-HT in the GIT.

5-hydroxytryptamine (5-HT; serotonin)

■ Originally called serotonin because it was first identified in serum and when injected increases blood pressure.
■ A monoamine.
■ Occurs in platelets and as a neurotransmitter and neuromodulator, notably in the brain and GIT.

Biosynthesis of 5-HT

■ Synthesis from dietary tryptophan.
■ Synthesis is regulated by tryptophan hydroxylase.

Currently perceived significance of 5-HT*

■ Neurotransmitter for several CNS pathways (*see* Figure 12.2).
■ High concentrations in GIT enteric neuronal plexus and epithelial enterochromaffin cells.
■ High concentrations in platelets with implications for mediation of platelet aggregation.
■ Mediation of smooth muscle contraction in the bronchi and uteri.

---

* A constantly fluid and changing area of pharmacology, due mainly to rapid advances in 5-HT receptor research.

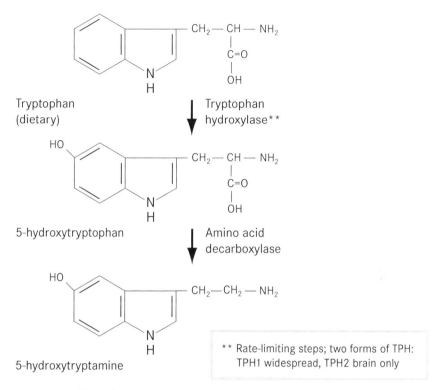

FIGURE 12.1 Biosynthesis of 5-hydroxytryptamine (5-HT; serotonin).

- Possible mediation of nociceptive nerve ending responsiveness to painful stimuli.
- Currently investigated for involvement in (for example):
  - appetite
  - aetiology of manic-depressive syndromes
  - aetiology of migraine
  - body temperature regulation
  - neuromodulator/neurotransmitter in the GIT*
  - mood, e.g. premenstrual tension, post-partum depression
  - aetiology of reward mechanisms
  - sexual behaviour
  - sleep-waking patterns and neural light/darkness driven rhythms
  - aetiology of infant cot death (possibly due to abnormal 5-HT neuron activity in the brainstem)
  - vomiting reflex.

---

* GIT: gastrointestinal tract.

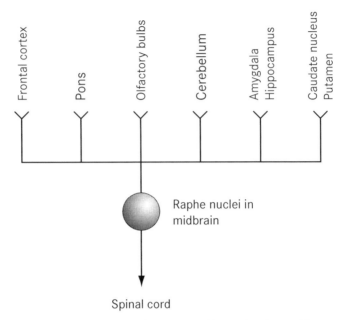

FIGURE 12.2 Ascending and descending central 5-H neural pathways (diagrammatic).

Clinical significance of 5-HT

■ Inspiration for development of drugs (for example):
  ▪ antidepressants, e.g. fluoxetine (Prozac® Dista)
  ▪ anti-emetics, e.g. ondansetron (Zofran® GSK)
  ▪ antipsychotics, e.g. ariprazole (Abilify® Bristol-Myers Squibb)
  ▪ for treatment of migraine, e.g. 5-HT1 agonist almotriptan
    (Almogran® Organon).

Release of 5-HT from neurones

■ Nerve impulse on 5-HT neurone stimulates release of 5-HT from:
  ▪ nerve terminal into synapse
  ▪ from varicosities along nerve.

Termination of action of 5-HT

■ Uptake of 5-HT into the nerve terminal by a serotonin-selective re-uptake transporter (SERT).
■ SERTs are members of the Na^+/Cl^+ transporter family.
■ SERTs are highly abundant in the mucosa of the GIT.
■ SERTs are targets for drugs which block their action and reduce their availability to endogenous* 5-HT (for example):

---

* *Endogenous*: produced by and occurring in the body.

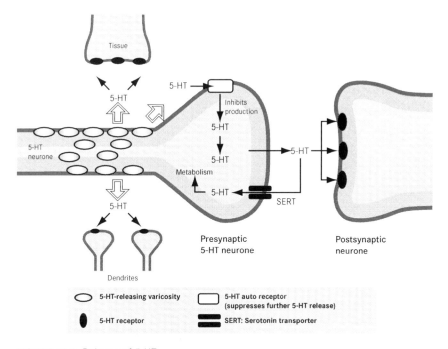

FIGURE 12.3 Release of 5-HT.

- SSRI* antidepressants such as fluoxetine
- tricyclic antidepressants, e.g. imipramine
- recreational drugs, e.g. 3,4-methylenedioxy-N-methylamphetamine (MMDA; 'Ecstasy').

Metabolism of 5-HT

- Conversion by monoamine oxidase (MAO) and aldehyde dehydrogenase to 5-hydroxyindoleacetic acid (5-HIAA) excreted in urine.

5-HT receptors

- Several 5-HT receptor subtypes have been discovered (see Table 12.1).
- 5-HT autoreceptors on presynaptic nerve inhibit further 5-HT release.

5-HT as a neurotransmitter and neuromodulator in the gastrointestinal tract (GIT)

- The GIT possesses a vast, virtually autonomous nervous system which employs almost every presently known neurotransmitter to serve sensory, motor and interneurone activity.

---

* SSRI: serotonin-selective re-uptake inhibitor.

TABLE 12.1 SECOND MESSENGERS: ALL ARE G PROTEIN-MEDIATED RECEPTORS EXCEPT FOR 5-HT$_3$, A LIGAND-GATED ION CHANNEL

SUBTYPE	LOCATION	MEDIATES	AGONISTS	ANTAGONISTS
5-HT$_{1A}$	CNS	Anxiety, feeding, sleep, thermogenesis	Buspirone	Ergotamine[1] Methiothepin[2] Spiperone Yohimbine
5-HT$_{1B}$	CNS Lungs	Behaviour, vasoconstriction	Ergotamine Sumatriptan[3]	Metergoline[4] Methiothepin
5-HT$_{1D}$	CNS	Vasoconstriction in CNS	Sumatriptan	Ergotamine Metergoline Methiothepin
5-HT$_{2A}$	CNS Vascular smooth muscle platelets	Learning, neuronal excitation, vasoconstriction or dilatation, platelet aggregation	LSD DOI (a 5-HT receptor agonist)	Cyproheptadine[5] Pizotifen[6] Ketanserin[7]
5-HT$_{2B}$	Smooth muscle of stomach	Smooth muscle contraction	LSD DOI α-methyl-5-HT	Yohimbine
5-HT$_{2C}$	CNS Choroid plexus	Mediates CSF secretion	LSD α-methyl-5-HT	Agomelatine[8]
5-HT$_3$	CNS Peripheral nerves	Anxiety, emesis[9] Neuronal excitation	α-methyl-5-HT	Odansetron[10] Mirtazapine[11] Renzapride[12]

SUBTYPE	LOCATION	MEDIATES	AGONISTS	ANTAGONISTS
5-HT$_4$	CNS GIT	Neuronal excitement Enhances GIT motility	Renzapride Metoclopramide[13] 5-methoxytryptamine	
5-HT$_{5A}$	CNS Ganglia	Possible role in arterial chemoreception Modulation of exploratory behaviour	LSD	
5-HT$_6$	CNS	Possible modulator of CNS cholinergic function Possible role in learning and memory	LSD	
5-HT$_7$	Widespread, e.g. CNS, GIT			

1. Ergotamine: Naturally occurring alkaloid extracted from ergot.
2. Methiothepin: A non-selective 5-HT receptor antagonist.
3. Sumatriptan: Drug introduced to treat migraine.
4. Metergoline: A derivative of ergot alkaloids; used to lower prolactin levels.
5. Cyproheptadine: A drug used as an antihistamine, occasionally for migraine and in the treatment of Cushing's disease.
6. Pizotifen: An antihistamine also used to treat migraine and cluster headaches.
7. Ketanserin: A drug being investigated for treatment of Raynaud's phenomenon (icy fingers in (e.g.) scleroderma).
8. Agomelatine: A newer anxiolytic and antidepressant.
9. Emesis: Vomiting.
10. Odansetron: An anti-emetic.
11. Mirtazapine: An antidepressant.
12. Renzapride: Used for constipation and irritable bowel syndrome.
13. Metoclopramide: Used to treat nausea and vomiting.

- These neurotransmitters mediate reflex responses and regulation of GIT motility and secretory activity.
- Most of the body's 5-HT is synthesised and employed in the human GIT.
- Most bowel 5-HT is synthesised by and stored in epithelial enterochromaffin cells.*
- Important physiological and pharmacological actions of 5-HT in the gut include:
  - mediation of peristalsis through increased contractility of GIT smooth muscle and increased motility
  - perhaps some modulation of secretory activity.

Chapter 12 Quiz

ANSWER T (TRUE) OR F (FALSE)

1. 5-HT occurs mainly in liver, CNS and gut. ☐
2. 5-HT is synthesised from dietary tryptophan. ☐
3. Synthesis is regulated by tyrosine hydroxylase. ☐
4. 5-HT is a CNS neurotransmitter mediating, (for example):
   Sleep-waking patterns. ☐
   Brain reward pathways. ☐
   Vomiting reflex. ☐
   Mood. ☐
   Migraine. ☐
   Body temperature regulation. ☐
5. 5-HT action is terminated by postsynaptic uptake. ☐
6. SERTs are targets for drugs that enhance 5-HT action at the synapse. ☐
7. 5-HT is metabolised to 5-hydroxyindole acetic acid, excreted in the urine. ☐
8. 5-HT autoreceptors on postsynaptic cells promote further synthesis of 5-HT. ☐
9. 5-HT is a relatively unimportant neurotransmitter and modulator in the GIT. ☐

---

* Enterochromaffin cells: endocrine epithelial cells of the GIT which store, for example, 5-HT or histamine in granules, and which often stain with salts of silver or chromium.

13 Eiconasoids

Learning objectives ■ A definition of eiconasoids ■ Some pharmacologically important eiconasoids ■ Prostaglandin receptors ■ Examples of drugs that intervene in the eiconasoid system

Learning objectives
- Be familiar with the different eiconasoids covered here and their receptors.
- Study the flow diagram for biosynthesis of the eiconasoids.
- Know that NSAIDs, including aspirin, work by inhibiting the COX-2 enzyme.
- Be aware of the protective effect of prostacyclin by inhibiting platelet aggregation.
- Know that thromboxane promotes platelet aggregation.
- Be acquainted with the names of drugs that block interleukin action.

A definition of eiconasoids
A collective term for compounds derived from 20-carbon fatty acids.

Some pharmacologically important eiconasoids
- Leukotrienes, (for example):
  - LTA4: Converted to LTB4
  - LTB4: Chemotactic* influence on migrating neutrophils
  - LTC4
  - LTD4
  - LTE4
  - LTF4

  Cystinyl leukotrienes: mediators of bronchoconstriction, increased capillary permeability and fast hypersensitivity responses
- Prostanoids, (for example):
  - prostaglandins, (for example):
    - PgD_2: evidence for involvement in rapid eye movement sleep, muscle contraction and relaxation, CNS trophic factor and neuromodulator; bronchoconstriction and airways remodelling
    - PgE_2: involved in uterine function, especially in implantation and parturition; contributes to tissue oedema, pain, and cytokine production in inflamed tissues; maintenance of gastric mucosal integrity; maintenance of glomerular filtration and renal blood flow

---

* Chemotaxis is the movement of cells in response to a chemical stimulus, here LTB4.

- ◆ PgF2α: mediates pain and inflammation (*see* aspirin, p. 164); protects against coagulation in endothelial tissue; involved in mammalian reproduction.
- ▌ prostacyclin (PgI$_2$):
  - ◆ prevents platelet aggregation, dilates arterioles.
- ▌ thromboxane:
  - ◆ TXA$_2$; produced by activated platelets; promotes platelet aggregation; vasoconstrictor; hypertensive (raised blood pressure); prothrombotic.

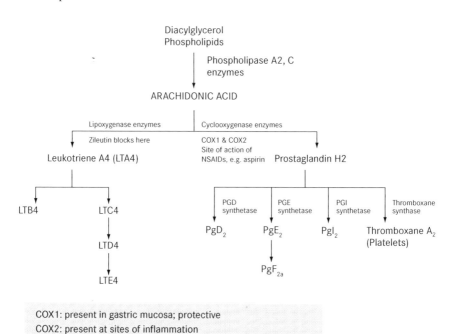

FIGURE 13.1 Summary of eiconasoid synthesis.

Prostaglandin receptors

- ▨ At least nine types named after the Pg that binds them:
  - ▌ DP-1 (for example) Prostaglandin D1 binds – DP-1
  - ▌ DP-2
  - ▌ EP-2
  - ▌ EP-4
  - ▌ IP
  - ▌ EP-1
  - ▌ EP-3
  - ▌ FP
  - ▌ TP.

Examples of drugs that intervene in the eiconasoid system

- Aspirin: blocks COX enzymes (*see* p. 164).
- NSAIDs: block COX enzymes, e.g. celecoxib (*see* p. 164).
- Prostacyclin, e.g. epoprostenol, for treatment of pulmonary hypertension and prevention of platelet aggregation.
- Leukotriene-modifying drugs, (for example):
  - zileuton blocks lipoxygenase enzyme activity and is a potential asthma treatment drug
  - montelukast and zafirlukast are used to treat asthma and block leukotriene receptor LTD4, and may inhibit expression of LTC4 receptors in bronchial tissue.

Chapter 13 Quiz

ANSWER T (TRUE) OR F (FALSE)

1. *Eiconasoids* is a collective term for 20-carbon fatty acids. ☐
2. Eiconasoids include prostanoids, leukotrienes and thromboxane. ☐
3. Prostaglandins:
   Are derived from arachidonic acid. ☐
   Mediate pain and inflammation. ☐
   Are involved in the process of implantation in the uterus. ☐
   Actions are blocked by paracetamol. ☐
4. Leukotrienes:
   Are important mediators of bronchial constriction. ☐
   Are synthesised through the action of cyclooxegenase enzymes. ☐
   Mediate increased capillary permeability. ☐
   Mediate fast hypersensitivity responses. ☐
   Inhibit chemotaxis. ☐
5. LTC4, LTD4 and LTE4 are cystinyl leukotrienes. ☐
6. Prostaglandin PGD_2 mediates bronchoconstriction, for example. ☐
7. PGE_2 enhances gastric mucosa breakdown. ☐
8. $PGF_2\alpha$ mediates pain and inflammation. ☐
9. Aspirin blocks prostaglandin production. ☐
10. Prostacyclin (PGI_2) inhibits platelet aggregation. ☐
11. Prostacyclin is used to treat pulmonary hypertension. ☐
12. Leukotriene-modifying drugs are used to treat asthma. ☐

14 Peptides and proteins as drugs ('biological' drugs)*

Learning objectives ■ Mini glossary ■ Protein biosynthesis summary ■ Mechanism of action of a biologic drug ■ Examples of polypeptide and protein drugs ■ Some problems with peptides and proteins as drugs

Learning objectives
■ Know what is meant by biological drugs and be able to give examples of them.

Mini glossary
■ Amino acid: building block of proteins, consisting of an amino group linked to a carboxyl group, e.g. Alanine: CH3-CH(NH2)-COOH.
■ Chimaeric: here describes a molecule produced using and made from biological material from more than one species.
■ DNA: deoxyribonucleic acid.
■ Biological (biologic) drug: therapeutic agent produced from biological starting material, e.g. an antibody, usually targeting a specific biological mediator, e.g. TNF-α[†], or process, e.g. angiogenesis.[‡]
■ EPo: erythropoietin.
■ Monoclonal antibodies: a population of antibodies produced by a single B cell clone that are therefore genetically identical to each other.
■ Peptide bond: chemical bond between an amino group of one molecule with the carboxyl group of another; how polypeptides and proteins are formed.
■ Polypeptide: chain of amino acids linked by peptide bonds.[§]
■ Protein: macromolecular polypeptide consisting of α-amino acids linked by peptide bonds, which has a biological function.
■ Protein structure:
　■ primary structure: amino acid sequence of the protein
　■ secondary structure: regular repeats of local structures determined by hydrogen bonding, e.g. the α-helix

---

* In the USA, they are termed 'biologic' drugs.
† TNF-α is tumour necrosis factor-alpha.
‡ Angiogenesis is development of new blood vessels (essential for tumour growth).
§ For polypeptides, some authorities put the upper limit at 50 amino acids.

- tertiary structure: protein shape determined by folding
- quaternary structure: structure determined by arrangement of protein subunits.
- RNA: ribonucleic acid.

Protein biosynthesis summary

1 Genetic transcription of mRNA.
2 Ribosomal translation of mRNA into protein strand.
3 Folding of protein into a tertiary structure predetermined through the composition and sequence of the constituent amino acids.
4 Combination of various subunit proteins to form the quaternary structure, e.g. haemoglobin is composed of 4 subunit proteins.

Mechanism of action of a biologic drug

1 The drug (e.g. Infliximab) is injected into the bloodstream.
2 The inflammatory mediator, e.g. TNF-α, binds to the TNF-α-binding site that has been incorporated into the Fab arm.
3 TNF-α is unable to bind to its receptor on cells that mediate the inflammatory response.

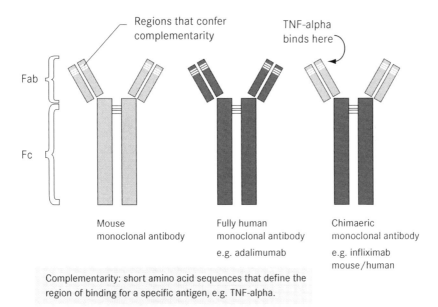

Complementarity: short amino acid sequences that define the region of binding for a specific antigen, e.g. TNF-alpha.

FIGURE 14.1 Biological drug structure.

Examples of polypeptide and protein drugs[*]

- Abciximab (ReoPro®; Lilly):
  - *nature of drug*: derived from Fab fragments of an immunoglobulin which targets the glycoprotein IIb/IIIa receptor on the platelet membrane
  - *action:* blocks platelet aggregation
  - *use*: procedures e.g. angioplasty.[†]
- Erythropoietin (EPo):[‡]
  - *nature of drug*: protein produced by the kidney when blood oxygen levels fall
  - *action*: stimulates red blood cell production in bone marrow
  - *use*: treatment of anaemia.
- Etanercept (Enbrel®; Wyeth):
  - *nature of drug*: a combination of two soluble human TNF receptors linked to an Fc portion of an IgG1, thus effectively producing an antibody to TNF-α
  - *action*: blocks TNF-α
  - *uses*: treatment of rheumatoid arthritis (RA) and psoriasis.
- Growth hormone:
  - *nature of drug*: naturally occurring but now also chemically synthesised hormone that promotes body growth
  - *action*: promotes body growth
  - *uses*: GH deficiency in adults and children; chronic renal insufficiency, Prader-Willi syndrome; Turner's syndrome.
- Infliximab (Remicade®; Schering-Plough):
  - *nature of drug*: a chimaeric monoclonal antibody
  - *action*: blocks TNF-α availability to tissues by binding it
  - *uses*: Crohn's disease, RA.
- Insulin:
  - *nature of drug*: naturally occurring but now chemically synthesised polypeptide hormone normally secreted from pancreatic islet cells; now produced by recombinant DNA technology
  - *action*: controls blood glucose levels, mainly by promoting glucose uptake into tissues
  - *use*: diabetes.

---

[*] Not comprehensive and the list is expanding fast; this is just a sample and more biological drugs are dealt with in the appropriate chapter.
[†] Angioplasty is surgical repair of blood vessels, usually arteries.
[‡] EPO is used illegally by some athletes to enhance performance.

- Interferons:[*]
  - *nature of drug*: group of proteins produced by cells under viral attack
  - *actions*: interfere with viral replication
  - *uses*: notably multiple sclerosis.
- Oxytocin:
  - *nature of drug*: peptide hormone released from the posterior pituitary gland
  - *actions*: suckling reflex; milk ejection; uterine contractions
  - *uses*: labour induction; stimulate breast-feeding; increase milk induction; (veterinary mainly); oxytocin receptor antagonists prevent premature labour, e.g. atosiban.
- Trastuzumab (Herceptin®; Genentech):
  - *nature of drug*: genetically engineered humanised monoclonal antibody
  - *action*: binds to the extracellular domain of the human epidermal growth factor receptor 2 [HER2/neu (ErbB2) on tumour cells] and arrests the G1 phase of the cell cycle; it also inhibits angiogenesis
  - *use*: breast cancer; in UK licensed as monotherapy for use in metastatic breast cancer which over-expresses HER2 receptors.
- Vaccines.
- Vasopressin and analogues of vasopressin:
  - *actions*: promotion of water re-uptake in renal collecting ducts; vasoconstriction; conservation of water and salt
  - *uses*: pituitary diabetes insipidus; bleeding form oesophageal varices.

Some problems with peptides and proteins as drugs

- Antibody generation in patients, i.e. immunogenic potential.
- Purification problems.
- Instability.
- Production may use non-human constituents of the final product.
- Need for parenteral administration, in some cases in the clinic.
- Adverse effects.
- Production and storage problems.
- Patient compromisation, e.g. some products suppress immune function.
- Cost to the NHS and the patient.

---

[*] Highly simplified here.

Chapter 14 Quiz

ANSWER T (TRUE) OR F (FALSE)

1. A chimaeric drug is constructed from more than one species. ☐
2. Monoclonal antibodies are derived from a single B cell clone. ☐
3. Erythropoietin stimulates white cell production. ☐
4. Polypeptides and proteins are formed via peptide bonds. ☐
5. TNF-α is a target for biological drugs. ☐
6. Abciximab is used to treat rheumatoid arthritis. ☐
7. Erythropoietin is used to treat anaemia. ☐
8. Etanercept is used to treat rheumatoid arthritis. ☐
9. Synthetic growth hormone is used preferentially.* ☐
10. Interferons are produced by cells under bacterial attack. ☐
11. Trastuzumab is used to treat metastatic breast cancer. ☐
12. Vasopressin is used to treat diabetes mellitus. ☐
13. Peptides and proteins as drugs may present problems involving:
    Purification. ☐
    Compromising patient immunity to infection. ☐
    Immunogenic potential of the drug. ☐
    Adverse effects. ☐
    Administration of the drug. ☐
    Production and storage. ☐
14. The quaternary structure of a protein is the amino acid sequence. ☐

* To avoid dangers of contamination with, for example, HIV.

15 Systems targeted by drugs

Systems targeted by drugs ■ Other uses of drugs ■ Drug interactions and drug toxicity ■ Special considerations when prescribing drugs ■ Legal and other issues

Systems targeted by drugs
- Blood.
- Cardiovascular system.
- Endocrine system.
- Immune system.
- Gastrointestinal system.
- Genito-urinary system.
- Musculoskeletal system and joints.
- Nervous system:
  - central nervous system (CNS)
  - peripheral nervous system (PNS).
- Respiratory system.
- Skin.
- Special senses:
  - eyes
  - ears.

Other uses of drugs
- Anaesthesia.
- Infection.
- Malignancy.
- Nutrition.
- Obstetrics.

DRUG INTERACTIONS AND DRUG TOXICITY
Special considerations when prescribing drugs
- Patient status: neonatal, aged.
- Organ status: liver, kidney.
- Immunocopetence.
- Pregnancy.

Legal and other issues

- Controlled drugs.
- Drug misuse.
- Pharmacoeconomics.
- Pharmacovigilance.
- Training and specialist skills.

16 Diuretics

Learning objectives

- Be able to list the classes of the diuretics given here.
- Be able describe the nature and use of mannitol.
- Be ready to give examples of the various classes of diuretics presented here, with uses, adverse effects, precautions and contraindications, where given.

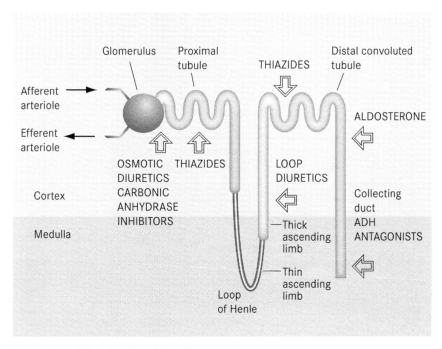

FIGURE 16.1 Sites of action of diuretics.

Diuretics

Diuretics are drugs which promote the flow of urine.

- Uses include:
  - ascites due to liver failure
  - cirrhosis of the liver
  - heart failure
  - hypertension
  - oliguria (poor urination) caused by kidney failure
  - peripheral and pulmonary oedema
  - renal disease.

Classes of diuretics covered here

- Osmotic diuretics.
- Carbonic anhydrase inhibitors.
- Loop diuretics.
- Thiazides.
- Potassium-sparing diuretics.

OSMOTIC DIURETICS

MANNITOL

- Is a large molecular weight sugar.
- Is administered IV.
- Increases plasma osmolality in the bloodstream, thus drawing water and salts from the tissues into the blood.
- Is filtered into the urine in the glomerulus.
- Increases the osmotic pressure in the filtered urine, drawing water and salts through the proximal tubule membrane into the urine and thus increases urine flow.
- Is often mixed with sodium bicarbonate to counteract its slight acidity in solution.

Uses of mannitol include

- Maintenance of an adequate urine flow during cardiovascular surgery.
- Treatment of cerebral oedema.
- Treatment of glaucoma.
- Treatment of kidney failure.

Adverse effects of mannitol include

- Electrolyte and fluid imbalances.
- Sensation of chill.
- Fever.

- Thrombophlebitis and inflammation on extravasation (escape into tissues during infusion).

Contraindications of mannitol include
- Severe dehydration.
- Anuria secondary to kidney disease.
- Pulmonary oedema or congestion.

CARBONIC ANHYDRASE INHIBITORS
ACETAZOLAMIDE
- Causes diuresis by increasing urinary bicarbonate.
- Useful for aspirin poisoning (aspirin is a weak acid, therefore more ionised in alkaline urine and more quickly eliminated).
- Is a weak diuretic; action is self-limiting.
- Is used mainly to treat glaucoma and as a prophylaxis against mountain sickness.
- Is used together with other drugs to treat epilepsy.
- May cause skin rashes and drowsiness (don't drive or operate dangerous machinery).
- Requires regular blood cell counts.

Precautions include
- Electrolyte imbalance.
- Emphysema.
- Liver disease.
- Pulmonary obstruction.

Contraindications include
- Adrenal failure.
- Chronic non-congestive glaucoma.
- Pregnancy; breast-feeding (may pass into breast milk).
- Severe hepatic or renal problems.
- Sulphonamide allergies.

THIAZIDES (AND RELATED COMPOUNDS)
- Are mainly derivatives of benzothiadiazine, hence the name – thiazides.
- Are of moderate potency as diuretics.
- Act at the beginning of the distal convoluted tubule to inhibit Cl⁻ reabsorption.

Include

- Bendroflumethiazide.
- Chlortalidone (thiazide-related).
- Hydrochlorothiazide.
- Indapamide.
- Metolazone.
- Xipamide.

Uses include

- Management of essential hypertension (act as a vasodilators).
- Treatment for mild to moderate heart failure (bendroflumethiazide – short-acting).
- Treatment for oedema (chlortalidone – longer duration than bendroflumethiazide.

Adverse effects include

- Electrolyte disturbances generally.
- Gout.
- Hypokalaemia (lowered plasma K^+).
- Hyperglycaemia (can exacerbate diabetes mellitus).
- Impotence.
- Photosensitivity.
- Postural hypotension.
- Raised cholesterol.

Precautions include

- Gout.
- Diabetes.
- SLE (can exacerbate SLE).
- Breast-feeding (thiazides may pass into breast milk).

Contraindications include

- Addison's disease.
- Hypercalcaemia.
- Hyponatraemia (lowered blood sodium).
- Lowered blood Mg^{2+}.
- Symptomatic hyperuricaemia.

LOOP DIURETICS

- Are the most potent of the diuretics.
- Are so-called because:
  - they inhibit Na^+ and Cl^- reabsorption in the thick part of the ascending loop of Henle by blocking the Cl^--binding site, which results in large volumes of hypotonic urine being presented to the distal tubules and the collecting ducts, thus reducing the osmotic 'pulling power' of the urine in the distal tubules and collecting ducts.

Uses include

- Treatment of pulmonary oedema due to left ventricular failure.
- Treatment of hypertension.
- Treatment of oliguria caused by renal failure.

Examples of loop diuretics

- Bumetanide.
- Furosemide (frusemide). ⎤ Similar onset (1 hour) and diuresis is complete within 6 hours
- Torasemide. ⎦

Adverse effects of loop diuretics (vary with individual drugs; some effects here)

- Bone marrow depression (patients should be monitored for this while on these drugs).
- Loss of cations especially, Na^+, K^+, Mg^{2+}. ⎤ Hypokalaemia is potentially fatal if patients are also on digoxin
- Deafness (especially with furosemide and bumetanide). ⎦
- Hyperuricaemia and gout.
- Pancreatitis with larger doses.
- Photosensitivity.
- Temporary elevation of plasma triglycerides and cholesterol.
- Skin rashes.
- Refractory oedema in congestive heart failure with inappropriate use of high dose loop diuretics, especially with high dietary Na^+ intake. It may be appropriate to lower the Na^+ intake and the dose of the loop diuretic and use in conjunction with a distally active diuretic, e.g. a thiazide (consult a specialist).

Precautions and contraindications with loop diuretics

- Precautions include:
  - hypotension
  - benign prostatic hyperplasia
  - kidney disease

▌ pregnancy.
▪ Contraindications include:
  ▌ liver cirrhosis with a precomatose state
  ▌ renal failure with anuria.

POTASSIUM-SPARING DIURETICS

Aldosterone antagonists
▪ Spironolactone. ⎤⎯ Block the action of aldosterone (the salt-retaining
▪ Eplerenone. ⎦ adrenocortical hormone) at its receptor in the distal tubule

Others
▪ Amiloride.
▪ Triamterine.

Mechanism note: generally, diuretics that work in the distal tubule and collecting ducts are less likely to cause significant K^+ loss.

ALDOSTERONE ANTAGONISTS

▪ Spironolactone.
▪ Eplerenone.

Clinical uses include
▪ Ascites and oedema due to liver cirrhosis.
▪ Primary hyperaldosteronism.
▪ Left ventricular problems after heart failure (eplerenone).

Clinical note: Do NOT give potassium supplements with potassium-sparing drugs.

Chapter 16 Quiz

ANSWER T (TRUE) OR F (FALSE)

1. Mannitol is useful in surgery to maintain renal function. ☐
2. Mannitol increases the osmolality of urine. ☐
3. Carbonic anhydrase inhibitors decrease urinary bicarbonate. ☐
4. Acetazolamide may be used to treat aspirin poisoning. ☐
5. Thiazides act at the glomerulus to enhance chloride excretion. ☐
6. Thiazide-like drugs include chlortalidone. ☐
7. Thiazides have moderate diuretic potency. ☐
8. Thiazides may be used to manage mild to moderate heart failure. ☐
9. Adverse effects of thiazides include hypoglycaemia. ☐
10. Thiazides are contraindicated in Addison's disease. ☐
11. Loop diuretics:

    Block Cl^- reabsorption in the glomerulus. ☐

    Result in small volumes of hypertonic urine presented to the tubules. ☐
12. Loop diuretics include bumetanide and furosemide. ☐
13. Loop diuretics are used for hypertension. ☐
14. Loop diuretics can cause bone marrow suppression. ☐
15. Spirinolactone blocks aldosterone action in the adrenal gland. ☐
16. Clinical uses of spirinolactone include oedema of liver cirrhosis. ☐
17. Thiazide diuretics are contraindicated in patients with gout. ☐

17 Drugs and the heart I: heart failure[*]

Learning objectives
- Be able to discuss briefly the difference between the normal and diseased heart with respect to congestive heart failure – know what Starling's Law states.
- Be able to list the important consequences of heart failure for the patient.
- Be able to list the six main classes of drugs used to treat heart failure.
- Know some examples and be able to list briefly their effects, mechanism of action given here and some adverse effects.

Mini glossary
- Afterload: resistance caused by the arterial pressure against which the heart has to pump.
- Cardiac output: volume of blood pumped by the heart per minute.
- Heart rate: the number of heart beats per minute.
- Preload: back pressure in the venous circulation which fills the heart and stretches the heart muscle.
- Stroke volume: the volume of blood pumped from the left ventricle in a single contraction of the heart.

The healthy heart
- Is a powerful pump driving blood with sufficient power and regularity to:
  - ensure adequate perfusion of tissues with blood at rest and during exercise
  - facilitate efficient return of blood to the heart.
- Beats autonomously and is also regulated by the sympathetic and parasympathetic nervous systems.

---

[*] Also called congestive heart failure.

- Obeys Starling's Law: the greater the diastolic volume, the greater the force of contraction. Or, the degree of cardiac muscle fibre contraction is a function of initial fibre length:
  - blood is not allowed to dam up in veins
  - more blood can be supplied per minute during exercise.
- Can respond to increased demand through exercise etc, by supplying blood to the tissues faster.

The diseased heart

- Does not obey Starling's Law, i.e. cannot respond to increased demand by supplying more blood.
- Becomes enlarged due to inadequate emptying of the ventricles.
- Has progressively thicker and stiffer vessel walls.

Some causes of heart failure

- Anaemia.
- Hypertension.
- Mitral regurgitation.*
- Some infections.
- Dysrthmias.
- Myocardial infarction.
- Pulmonary embolism.
- Thyrotoxicosis.

Important consequences of heart failure for the patient

- Patient cannot exercise effectively.
- Potential organ damage, e.g. kidney, which cannot filter properly.
- Oedema in peripheral tissues especially lungs and ankles, due to increased preload,, i.e. back pressure pushing fluid out of capillaries into the tissues.
- Increased risk of mortality.

Treatment of heart failure

- Aims to restore cardiac ability to obey Starling's Law.
- Aims to decrease the heart's workload.
- Aims to reduce the preload.
- Aims to reduce oedema.
- Improves tolerance to physical exertion.
- Aims to reduce mortality.
- Employs six different type of drug:
  - ACE inhibitors (ACE: Angiotensin-Converting Enzyme); ACE inhibitors suppress the renin-angiotensin-aldosterone system
  - angiotensin-II receptor blockers
  - β-blockers (*see* p. 104) to reduce sympathetic tone to the heart, which reduces probability of morbidity and mortality

---

* Mitral regurgitation: leakage of blood back into the left atrium from the ventricle.

- diuretics (*see* p. 79) to mobilise oedema water through increased excretion of water and salt
- vasodilators, e.g. sodium nitroprusside and glyceryl trinitrate, to reduce venous pressure
- drugs to restore Starling's Law, notably digoxin (now used more for arrhythmias; *see* p. 101).

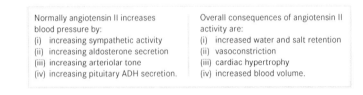

Normally angiotensin II increases blood pressure by:	Overall consequences of angiotensin II activity are:
(i) increasing sympathetic activity	(i) increased water and salt retention
(ii) increasing aldosterone secretion	(ii) vasoconstriction
(iii) increasing arteriolar tone	(iii) cardiac hypertrophy
(iv) increasing pituitary ADH secretion.	(iv) increased blood volume.

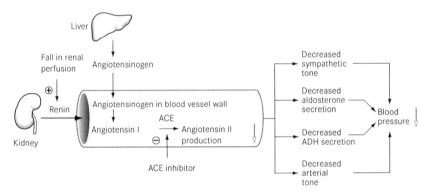

FIGURE 17.1 ACE inhibitor action.

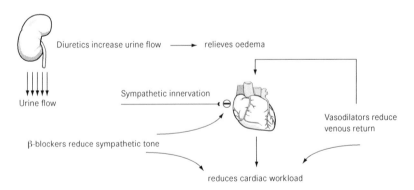

FIGURE 17.2 β-blockers, diuretics and vasodilators reduce cardiac workload in heart failure.

ACE inhibitors

- Captopril.
- Enalapril.
- Imidapril (Tanatril® Trinitry).
- Moexipril (Perdix® Schwartz).
- Quinapril.
- Trandolapril (Gopten® Abbott).
- Cilazapril (Vascase® Roche).
- Fosinopril.
- Lisinopril.
- Perindopril (Conversyl® Servier).
- Ramipril.

Mechanism of action: inhibition of angiotensin-converting enzyme (ACE; *see* Figure 17.1).

Effects of ACE inhibitors

- Increase cardiac output.
- Increase stroke volume.
- Lower the renovascular resistance.
- Increase venous capacitance (increased venous pooling).
- Increase sodium and water excretion.

Clinical use of ACE inhibitors

- Uses include:
  - heart failure
  - hypertension (*see* p. 147)
  - left ventricular problems
  - diabetes to reduce risk of peripheral neuropathies (*see* p. 145)
  - prevention of cardiovascular disease.
- Administration: oral tablets, usually together with a diuretic (*see* p. 90).

Adverse effects and precautions with ACE inhibitors

- Kidney:
  - ACE inhibitors can cause renal failure in patients with bilateral renal artery stenosis (narrowing of the lumen); use with caution in patients with renovascular disease. Check renal function before prescribing ACE inhibitors
  - may be dangerous if used concomitantly with diuretics: with initial doses, can cause a rapid hypotension in volume-depleted patients, whose Na^+ is low; blood pressure must be monitored in these patients after the first dose of ACE.
- Contraindications:
  - pregnancy
  - patients hypersensitive to ACE inhibitors
  - do not use in patients with suspected or known renovascular disease.

- Adverse effects (not comprehensive):
  - dry, persistent cough ⎤
  - angioedema (swellings beneath skin, ⎬ Caused because ACE inhibitors
    often around eyes and lips) ⎪ block kinin (e.g. bradykinin)
  - skin rashes ⎦ breakdown as well
  - upper respiratory tract symptoms, e.g. rhinitis, sore throat
  - blood dyscrasias (any abnormality within the blood system)
  - CNS effects, e.g. dizziness.

Angiotensin-II receptor blockers

- Candesartan (Amias® Takeda).
- Eprosartan (Teveten® Solvay).
- Irbesartan (Aprovel® Bristol-Myers Squibb/Sanofi-Synthelabo).
- Losartan potassium (Cozaar® MSD).
- Olmesartan (Olmetec® Sankyo).
- Telmisartan (Micardis® Boehringer Ingelheim).
- Valsartan (Diovan® Novartis).
- Mechanism:
  - blocks angiotensin-II at its AT1 receptor.
- Uses:
  - alternative to ACE inhibitors in patients with persistent cough.
- Adverse effects:
  - mainly mild; some angioedema reported; dizziness; hyperkalaemia.
- Precautions:
  - renovascular disease
  - aortic or mitral valve stenosis
  - elderly patients and patients already on diuretics; in these patients it is advisable to monitor plasma K^+.
- Contraindication:
  - pregnancy.

Diuretics

- Thiazides, e.g. bendroflumethiazide (also called bendrofluazide):
  - mechanism: inhibition of Na^+ and Cl^- transport in the cortical thick ascending limb and early distal tubule
  - use: together with ACE inhibitors or A-II receptor antagonists for patients with fluid overload
  - potential problems: retention of calcium and uric acid, therefore contraindicated in gout
  - limitations: ineffective if patients have severe heart failure and impaired renal function – use a loop diuretic instead (*see* below).

- Loop diuretics, e.g. furosemide (previously called frusemide):
  - mechanism: block the $Na^+/K^+/Cl^-$ co-transporter in the apical membrane of the thick ascending limb of the Loop of Henle
  - use: alone or together with a thiazide diuretic if indicated
  - potential problems: electrolyte imbalance with profound diuresis.
- Aldosterone antagonists, e.g. spironolactone:
  - mechanism: blocks the action of aldosterone at its receptor in the kidney
  - use: low dose for severe heart failure for patients already on a diuretic and an ACE inhibitor, as it may reduce mortality.
- Digoxin:
  - acts as diuretic only in heart failure because it improves cardiac output, which in turn mobilises oedema water and diuresis occurs; currently used more to treat certain dysrhythmias (*see* p. 101).

β-blockers
(*see also* p. 105)
- Bisoprolol.
- Carvedilol:
  - mechanism: reduces sympathetic influence on heart by blocking β-receptors; bisoprolol is more selective on cardiac $β_1$-receptors
  - uses: recently shown to reduce mortality in patients with left-ventricular systolic dysfunction and any form of stable heart failure
  - contraindications:[*] asthma (for all β-blockers) and uncontrolled heart failure.

Sodium nitroprusside
- Mechanism: dissolves to release the $[Fe(CN)_5NO]^{2-}$ metal nitrosyl complex, which is a potent venous and arterial dilator, thus reducing both pre- and afterload.
- Use: chronic heart failure and certain forms of hypertension.
- Adverse effects: reflect the sudden reduction in blood pressure, e.g. headache, syncope (fainting), dizziness, nausea and vomiting, palpitations.
- Contraindications: include severe vitamin B_{12} deficiency; compensatory hypertension and Leber's optic atrophy.[†]

---

[*] As with all contraindications, these are not comprehensive and will depend on the individual patient's condition.
[†] Loss of visual acuity and progressive blindness due to mitochondrial mutations.

Chapter 17 Quiz

ANSWER T (TRUE) OR F (FALSE)

1. Afterload is arterial resistance against which the heart has to pump. ☐
2. Preload is venous back pressure. ☐
3. The diseased heart responds to stretch with increased contractility. ☐
4. The diseased heart becomes enlarged. ☐
5. Heart failure may be caused by hypothyroidism. ☐
6. Patients with heart failure cannot exercise effectively. ☐
7. Oedema and kidney failure are associated with heart failure. ☐
8. Treatment aims to restore cardiac ability to obey Starling's Law. ☐
9. Treatment aims to increase the heart's workload. ☐
10. Treatment aims to decrease preload and oedema. ☐
11. ACE inhibitors block the breakdown of angiotensin-II. ☐
12. β-blockers help by increasing sympathetic tone to the heart. ☐
13. Diuretics help by reducing oedema water and salt. ☐
14. Vasodilators, e.g. nitroprusside, help by reducing preload. ☐
15. Digoxin restores the heart's ability to obey Starling's Law. ☐
16. ACE inhibitors are contraindicated with renovascular disease. ☐
17. Caution! ACE inhibitors potentiate diuretics. ☐
18. Thiazide diuretics are contraindicated in patients with gout. ☐
19. Loop diuretics block $Na^+/K^+/Cl^-$ reabsorption in the collecting ducts. ☐
20. β-blockers are contraindicated in asthmatic patients. ☐
21. β-blockers may reduce mortality in patients with left-ventricular systolic dysfunction. ☐

18 Drugs and the heart II: myocardial infarction (heart attack)

Learning objectives
- Be able to give a definition of myocardial infarction.
- Know the symptoms and early complications of a heart attack.
- Be able to give an account of the diagnosis and treatment strategies.

Mini glossary
- Angioplasty: insertion of a medical stent (splint placed inside a duct to maintain patency) or a balloon.
- Cardiopulmonary resuscitation: emergency chest compression and mouth-to-mouth ventilation (*see* Figure 18.4).
- ECG: electrocardiogram.
- Electrical cardioversion: conversion of abnormal cardiac rhythm to a normal rhythm using a defibrillator; cardioversion can also be achieved with drugs.
- Heart block: failure of conduction of the nerve impulse in cardiac tissue.
- Percutaneous coronary intervention (PCI): an invasive procedure to widen the narrowed coronary arteries, which is usually caused by build-up of cholesterol.
- Positive inotrope: an agent that increases the force and perhaps also the rate of cardiac contractions.
- LDL: low density lipoprotein.
- Myocardial infarction: death of heart muscle cells caused by interrupted blood supply, most usually in the left ventricle (*see* Figure 18.1).
- Pulmonary oedema: fluid accumulation in lung tissue.
- Streptokinase: an enzyme extracted from streptococcus that liquefies blood clots.
- Thrombolysis: dissolving a blood clot.
- Thrombus: blood clot.

- Ventricular fibrillation: rapid, irregular and uncoordinated ventricular twitching, resulting in death due to hypoxia unless treated in time.
- Ventricular tachycardia: rapid, regular heartbeat originating in the ventricle; dangerous because it may lead to ventricular fibrillation.

A definition of myocardial infarction

- Death of myocardial tissue, usually because of interruption of blood supply by a thrombus (blood clot), usually occurring in the left ventricular wall.

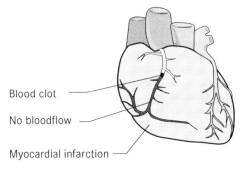

Blood clot

No bloodflow

Myocardial infarction

FIGURE 18.1 Myocardial infarction.

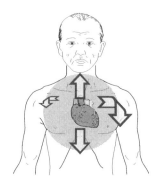

FIGURE 18.2 Radiation of pain of heart attack.

Some risk factors for myocardial infarction

- Ageing.
- Diabetes.
- Hyperlipoproteinaemia (raised LDL).
- Hypertension.
- Inactive lifestyle coupled with ill-advised diet.
- Obesity.

- Smoking.
- Social grouping (*see* Figure 18.3).*

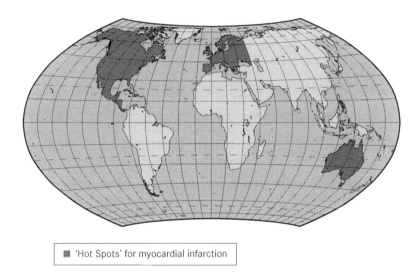

■ 'Hot Spots' for myocardial infarction

FIGURE 18.3 'Hot Spots' for myocardial infarction (approximation).

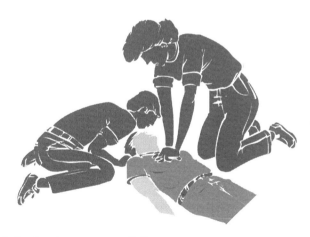

FIGURE 18.4 Cardiopulmonary resuscitation.

Symptoms of a heart attack

- Sudden, intense chest pain, often spreading into arms, particularly the left arm, and the throat.
- Breathlessness due to pulmonary oedema.

---

* Baldness in men and a so-called diagonal earlobe crease have been linked anecdotally to the risk of heart attack, but at present remain just that – anecdotal.

- Anxiety and sweating due to sympathetic activation.
- Sometimes no symptoms ('silent heart attack').
- Early complications include:
  - ventricular tachycardia, which may develop into ventricular fibrillation
  - heart block
  - ventricular fibrillation:
    - ◆ emergency electrical cardioversion needed
    - ◆ may need emergency cardiopulmonary resuscitation.

Diagnosis and treatment

- Diagnosis:
  - medical history
  - ECG.
- Treatment options (if no contraindications to thrombolysis):
  - oxygen
  - dispersible aspirin
  - IV morphine or diamorphine
  - streptokinase
  - heparin
  - if necessary IV dobutamine to provide inotropic support
  - amiodarone to treat arrhythmias
  - digoxin use is debatable but has been used in smaller doses as an inotrope in patients with chronic heart failure which is secondary to left ventricular systolic impairment; used in patients who are in sinus rhythm
  - fluid resuscitation to compensate for inadequate filling pressures.
- Percutaneous coronary intervention (PCI) – an alternative treatment to thrombolysis; involves:
  - angioplasty
  - drugs, including:
    - ◆ clopidogrel (Plavix®
      Bristol-Myers Squibb/Sanofi-Synthelabo)
    - ◆ GPIIb/IIIa receptor antagonists eptifibatide (Integrilin® GSK)
    - ◆ tirofiban (Aggrastat® MSD)
    - Platelet aggregation inhibitors (*see* p. 117)
    - ◆ heparin, an anticoagulant (*see* p. 124).
- Follow-up treatment after initial treatment includes:
  - β-blockers (*see* p. 104)
  - regular aspirin to inhibit platelet aggregation
  - a statin, which reduces plasma LDL (*see* p. 113)
  - ACE inhibitors (*see* p. 147).

Chapter 18 Quiz

ANSWER T (TRUE) OR F (FALSE)

1. Heart block is failure of impulse conduction in cardiac tissue. ☐

2. Cardiopulmonary resuscitation is emergency chest compression and mouth-to-mouth ventilation. ☐

3. Thrombolysis is dissolving of a blood clot. ☐

4. Risk factors for myocardial infarction include:

   Hypertension. ☐

   Anorexia. ☐

5. Ventricular tachycardia (VT) is an early complication of a heart attack. ☐

6. VT can develop into ventricular fibrillation unless treated. ☐

7. Symptoms of myocardial infarction include:

   Intense pain into arms and throat. ☐

   Breathlessness. ☐

   Anxiety and sweating. ☐

   Perhaps no symptoms. ☐

8. Diagnosis includes ECG and medical history. ☐

9. Pharmacological interventions include:

   Oxygen. ☐

   Dispersible aspirin. ☐

   Streptokinase. ☐

   IV diamorphine (heroin) or morphine. ☐

   Heparin. ☐

   Amiodarone. ☐

   Fluid resuscitation. ☐

10. Percutaneous coronary intervention is a procedure to widen coronary arteries. ☐

11. Platelet aggregation inhibitors include:

    Clopidogrel. ☐

    GPIIb/IIIa receptor antagonists. ☐

12. Follow-up treatment for myocardial infarction includes:

    Regular low-dose aspirin. ☐

    A statin. ☐

    ACE inhibitors. ☐

    β-blockers. ☐

19 Drugs and the heart III: antidysrhythmic drugs

Learning objectives ■ Normal cardiac rhythm ■ Arrhythmias ■ Automaticity
■ Re-entrant (circus) arrhythmias ■ Diagnosis ■ Treatment of arrhythmias:
antidysrhythmic drugs

Learning objectives
- Know the given factors controlling normal heart rhythm and be able to sketch quickly the main conduction pathways (*see* Figure 19.1).
- Be able to state briefly what arrhythmias are and their consequences for the patient.
- Know the definition of automaticity and of the meaning of re-entrant (circus) arrhythmias.
- Know the three main aims of treatment with antidysrhythmic drugs.
- Be aware of the main features of the Vaughan-Williams classification of antidysrhythmic drugs, with examples of drugs.
- Read through the examples of drugs and their uses, adverse effects, precautions and contraindications.

Normal cardiac rhythm
- Is controlled by the heart's pacemaker, the sino-atrial node (*see* Figure 19.1), which lies in the wall of the right atrium.
- Is also under the influence of autonomic inputs to the sino-atrial node (*see* pp. 34, 40, 99).
- Is achieved through the spread of electrical impulses through conducting tissues to the muscles of the atria and ventricles.

Arrhythmias
- Are deviations from the normal sinus rhythm of the heart.
- May be temporary physiological responses to the body's normal needs during, e.g. exercise or stress.
- May be:
  - pathologically induced through, e.g. damage to cardiac conducting tissue or the muscle, which can result in disturbances of conduction
  - of no apparent cause (idiopathic)
- May occur intermittently or continuously.

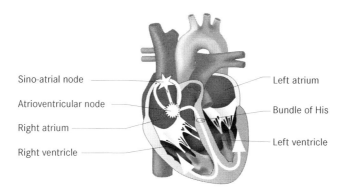

FIGURE 19.1 The heart nodes.

- Produce symptoms including:
  - breathlessness
  - chest pain
  - 'palpitations'.
- Are potentially life-threatening in some cases.
- May involve:
  - ectopic* beats, also called extrasystoles
  - fibrillation, which means rapid, uncoordinated beating or quivering of cardiac tissue, either in the atria, ventricles or both; both must be treated as medical emergencies
  - heart block, which is loss of co-ordination between the beating of the atria and ventricles, and which may be:
    - first degree heart block: conduction between atria and ventricles is delayed
    - second degree heart block: not all impulses generated in the atria reach the ventricles
    - third degree (complete) heart block: no impulses from the atria reach the ventricles, which beat at their intrinsic slow rate of about 25–45 beats per minute (normal HR is ~ 60–80 beats per minute)
  - tachycardia, which means speeding of the heart rate and can be dangerous;† it may lower blood pressure and cause dizziness and fainting; most tachycardias are not dangerous, but excessively fast beats can become fatal.

Automaticity

- Is a property of all cardiac muscle cells, which are capable of initiating an impulse on their own; this causes an ectopic focus.

---

* Ectopic in medicine means 'in the wrong place'; here meaning beats anywhere in the heart but the pacemaker.
† Normal sinus tachycardia is produced during the response of the heart to the demands of exercise.

- Can result in the establishment anywhere in the heart of a sustained ectopic beat.
- Is aggravated by sympathetic autonomic activity.

Re-entrant (circus) arrhythmias

- Are the establishment of an ectopic focus caused by tissue damage, which forces impulses to travel in a circle where the damage is (*see* Figure 19.2).
- Can cause:
  - atrial flutter, in atria, which is organised but extremely rapid beating, e.g. 25–300 beats per minute due to circus movement of impulses in the atria
  - supraventricular tachycardia, which is abnormally fast heartbeat; so-called because the tachycardia has its origins above the ventricles
  - ventricular tachycardia, in ventricles, when circus movement is in the ventricular muscle; potentially serious due to possibility of development to ventricular fibrillation, which is very fast uncoordinated flutters of the ventricles with disruption to blood ejection from the ventricles; is a potentially fatal emergency situation.

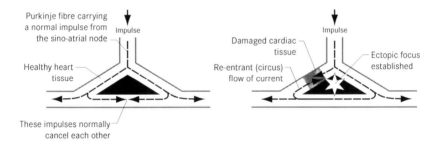

FIGURE 19.2 Re-entrant circuit.

Diagnosis*

- Depends mainly on the use of the ECG and interpretation of the traces obtained (*see* Figure 19.3).

Treatment of arrhythmias: antidysrhythmic drugs

- Are drugs designed mainly to slow the heart and to restore the normal rhythm by:
  - correcting abnormal pacemaker activity and/or
  - abnormal impulse propagation in the heart.

---

* There are very many different types of arrhythmias within the atria and ventricles, and are not dealt with here; the interested reader should consult more comprehensive texts.

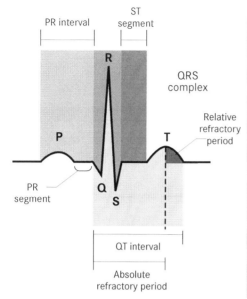

P wave: represents atrial depolarisation
QRS complex: represents ventricular depolarisation
T wave: represents ventricular recovery phase
Absolute refractory period = start of QRS complex to apex of T wave
Relative refractory period = second half of T wave

Interpretation of the ECG (not comprehensive):
• PR interval prolonged: perhaps heart block
• PR segment depressed: perhaps atrial damage
• Depressed ST segment may indicate coronary ischaemia
• Elevated ST segment may indicate MI
• Prolonged QT interval: prolonged (>0.44 seconds indicates danger of ventricular arrhythmia and sudden death)
• Drugs, e.g. Class IA antiarrhythmics, prolong the duration of the action potential

FIGURE 19.3 The ECG.

TABLE 19.1 VAUGHAN-WILLIAMS CLASSIFICATION OF ANTIDYSRHYTHMIC DRUGS (EXTENSIVELY MODIFIED OVER TIME)

CLASS OF DRUG	MECHANISM OF ACTION	EXAMPLES OF DRUGS
Class I Na^{2+} channel blockers		
1A	Prolong action potential	Procainamide, quinidine
1B	Shorten action potential	Lidocaine, mexiletine, phenytoin
1C	Depress rate of depolarisation	Flecainide, propafenone
Class II	β-blockers	Atenolol, esmolol, propranolol
Class III	K^+ channel blockers	Amiodarone, sotalol
Class IV	Ca^{2+}-channel L-type blockers**	Diltiazem, verapamil
Class V	Various other drugs	Adenosine, digoxin

** L-type Ca^{2+} channels mediate the prolonged Phase 2 plateau phase of the action potential in atrial, Purkinje, and ventricular cells.

- Have been classified:
  - according to their site of action as those treating:
    - supraventricular arrhythmias, e.g. verapamil
    - both supraventricular and ventricular arrhythmias, e.g. disopyramide
    - ventricular arrhythmias, e.g. lidocaine.

Antidysrhythmic drugs were most famously classified by Vaughan-Williams[*] according to their mechanism of action.

Class I

- Class IA, e.g. disopyramide, procainamide; block fast Na^+ channels and prolong the duration of the action potential (*see* Figure 19.3):
  - uses:
    - usually supraventricular tachycardia
    - ventricular arrhythmias
    - prevention of ventricular fibrillation
    - conversion of atrial fibrillation to normal sinus rhythm
  - precautions:[†]
    - not usually suitable for heart failure patients or any other condition which has weakened the heart
    - use of procainamide together with AV node blockers, e.g. digoxin may be advisable because procainamide alone promotes AV node conductivity and may speed up the ventricles.
- Class IB, e.g. lidocaine, mexiletine; Na^+-channel blockers that shorten the duration of the AP:
  - uses:
    - primarily treatment of life-threatening ventricular arrhythmias
    - lidocaine is used for emergencies especially following MI
  - precautions:[‡]
    - doses of lidocaine should be lowered in patients after cardiac surgery or with congestive heart failure
    - monitor blood pressure and ECG (*see* Figure 19.3).
- Class IC: these depress the rate of depolarisation (phase O of the action potential) and are the most powerful Na^+-channel blockers, e.g. flecainide, propafenone.
- Uses:[§]
  - flecainide:
    - paroxysmal supraventricular tachycardia

---

[*] Not entirely comprehensive but still useful (and employed).
[†] *See* the BNF for more comprehensive precautions.
[‡] *See* the BNF for more comprehensive precautions.
[§] Not comprehensive.

- ♦ prevention of paroxysmal atrial fibrillation
- ♦ prevention of suspected life-threatening ventricular tachycardias
- ♦ arrhythmias associated with the Wolff-Parkinson-White syndrome*
- ♦ has local anaesthetic effects.
- ▌ propafenone:
  - ♦ ventricular arrhythmias
  - ♦ paroxysmal atrial fibrillation or flutter
  - ♦ AV node-associated re-entrant paroxysmal tachycardias.
- ▓ Some reported adverse effects:
  - ▌ flecainide:
    - ♦ amnesia
    - ♦ confusion
    - ♦ dizziness, nausea, vomiting
    - ♦ hallucinations
    - ♦ lung inflammation (pneumonitis)
    - ♦ mental depression
    - ♦ photosensitivity
    - ♦ skin reactions
    - ♦ visual disturbances.
  - ▌ propafenone:
    - ♦ antimuscarinic effects, e.g. blurred vision, dry mouth
    - ♦ paradoxical arrhythmias
    - ♦ headache
    - ♦ hypotension.
- ▓ Precautions:†
  - ▌ patients with pacemakers
  - ▌ liver disease, especially with propafenone (liver-metabolised)
  - ▌ defects in atrial conduction (flecainide)
  - ▌ asthmatic patients (propafenone; β-blocking activity)
  - ▌ sinus or AV node dysfunction
  - ▌ heart failure
  - ▌ renal impairment with flecainide
  - ▌ patients on digoxin (monitor digoxin levels closely)
  - ▌ flecainide is excreted in milk.
- ▓ Contraindications:‡
  - ▌ flecainide:
    - ♦ asymptomatic ventricular ectopic beats or asymptomatic non-sustained ventricular tachycardia

---

* Wolff-Parkinson-White syndrome: an extra impulse conduction pathway in the heart that can cause arrhythmias.
† Not comprehensive.
‡ *See* BNF for more details.

+ previous history of MI
+ heart failure
+ patients with non-programmable pacemakers
+ abnormal left ventricular function.

  ▪ propafenone:
  + atrial conduction defects
  + AV block 2nd degree or greater
  + bundle branch block*
  + defects of atrial node function
  + electrolyte imbalances
  + postural hypotension in the elderly
  + severe bradycardia
  + severe obstructive pulmonary disease
  + uncontrolled congestive heart failure.

Class II: β-blockers *(see p. 105, Table 19.2)*

▪ Action:
  ▪ blockade of β_1-adrenoceptors in the heart, which reduces sympathetic tone.
▪ Uses in treatment of arrhythmias:
  ▪ management of supraventricular tachycardias following MI
  ▪ with digoxin to manage ventricular responses during atrial fibrillation.
▪ Adverse effects include:
  ▪ cold extremities
  ▪ fatigue.
▪ Precautions:
  ▪ previous history of hypersensitivity (danger of enhanced sensitivity to other allergens)
  ▪ any history of obstructive airways disease
  ▪ myasthenia gravis
  ▪ pregnancy and breast-feeding.
▪ Contraindications:[†]
  ▪ asthma
  ▪ heart failure that is unstable and poorly controlled
  ▪ hypotension
  ▪ patients with 2nd or 3rd degree heart block
  ▪ severe bradycardia.

---

* Bundle branch block: disruption of normal impulse flow through the nerve bundles to the Bundle of His or in the Bundle of His itself.
† Not comprehensive; *see* BNF for more details.

TABLE 19.2 RELATIVE SELECTIVITY OF β–ADRENOCEPTOR ANTAGONISTS

β-BLOCKING DRUG	RELATIVE AFFINITY FOR β_1-RECEPTOR
Bisoprolol	13.5
Betaxolol	6.8
Atenolol	4.7
Metoprolol	2.3
Carvedilol	0.2
Propranolol	0.1
Sotalol (also has Class 3 actions)	0.1
Timolol	<0.1

Note: A value <1 = selectivity for β_2-receptors; a value >1 = selectivity for β1-receptors.

Class III

These mainly block the K^+ channels, which prolongs the repolarisation phase of the action potential; Na^+ channels are unaffected, which means that conduction velocity is not decreased by class III drugs, e.g. amiodarone, sotalol (also Class II).

- Uses in treating arrhythmias:
    - amiodarone (use only under specialist supervision or in hospital)
    - administration is usually IV
    - atrial fibrillation and flutter
    - sustained ventricular tachycardia
    - resuscitation from ventricular fibrillation or pulseless tachycardia
    - prevention of recurrence of ventricular fibrillation
    - tachyarrhythmias associated with the Wolff-Parkinson-White syndrome.[*]
- Adverse effects:
    - very long half-life; steady-state plasma concentrations take a long time to be established; elimination is slow
    - thyroid disturbances (amiodarone contains iodine)
    - corneal micro deposits (common)
    - phototoxicity
    - skin rashes
    - pulmonary toxicity.

---

[*] Wolff-Parkinson-White syndrome: association of paroxysmal tachycardia (or atrial fibrillation) and pre-excitation, in which the electrocardiogram displays a short P-R interval and a wide QRS complex.

- Precautions:
  - chest X-ray, liver and thyroid function tests and plasma K^+ checked before treatment
  - use with caution after heart failure and in the elderly.
- Contraindications (unless absolutely essential to use, e.g. in cardiac arrest):
  - iodine sensitivity or thyroid disease
  - pregnancy and breast-feeding
  - sino-atrial heart block
  - sinus bradycardia[*]
  - don't use IV in cases of:
    - circulatory collapse
    - severe arterial hypotension
    - severe respiratory failure
  - don't give bolus[†] doses in:
    - cardiomyopathy
    - congestive heart failure.

Class IV

These block mainly Ca^{2+} L-type ion channels, e.g. verapamil, used to treat supraventricular tachycardias.
- Adverse effects include:
  - constipation
  - headache, nausea and vomiting
  - more rarely, skin reactions, gynaecomastia
  - gingival (gum) hyperplasia after prolonged use.
- Precautions are needed with:
  - first-degree AV block[‡]
  - patients on β-blockers
  - myocardial infarction (heart attack), especially in the acute phase
  - pregnancy and breast-feeding
  - liver-impaired patients.
- Contraindicated in patients with:
  - a history of heart attacks (myocardial infarction)
  - atrial flutter or fibrillation[§]
  - impaired left ventricular function

---

[*] Sinus rhythm with a resting heart rate of 60 beats/minute or less.
[†] Bolus: a single (sometimes large) dose of a drug.
[‡] First-degree AV block: abnormally slow (> 0.2 sec) for movement of impulse through the AV node, i.e. movement of the impulse from atria to ventricles is too slow.
[§] Atrial flutter: abnormally rapid but nevertheless regular contractions of the atria of the heart (± 250–350 contractions per minute); atrial fibrillation: irregular, poorly organised and rapid twitches or quivering of the atria.

▌ bradycardia, hypotension, sino-atrial block, 2nd and 3rd degree AV block*

▌ sick sinus syndrome†

▌ porphyria.

Class V: Adenosine and digoxin

▦ Digoxin:

  ▌ uses:

    ♦ formerly the mainstay for heart failure, but now used mainly for: atrial fibrillation and atrial flutter.

  ▌ mechanisms of action:

    ♦ digoxin blocks the Na^+/ATPase pump, resulting in inhibition of Ca^{2+} extrusion and increase Ca^{2+} stores in the sarcoplasmic reticulum

    ♦ digoxin slows the heart by enhancing vagal (parasympathetic) drive to the heart, thus slowing it down.

▦ Adverse effects include:‡

  ▌ nausea, vomiting, blurred vision (yellow haloes – a dangerous sign), dizziness, confusion and many more.

▦ Precautions:

  ▌ digoxin blood levels should be monitored during treatment

  ▌ hypokalaemia or low plasma Ca^{2+}; use with care if at all in patients who are hypokalaemic (low blood potassium); low blood K^+ or low blood Ca^{2+} enhance digoxin's toxicity

  ▌ renal disease: the kidneys are important in digoxin excretion; renal impairment can result in toxic effects from therapeutic doses of digoxin.

▦ Contraindications include:

  ▌ Wolff-Parkinson-White syndrome (*see* footnote p. 105)

  ▌ ventricular tachycardia or fibrillation

  ▌ intermittent complete heart block

  ▌ second degree AV block

  ▌ intermittent complete heart block

  ▌ pregnancy: effects of digoxin on the developing embryo and foetus are unknown; use only if necessary.

▦ Adenosine

▦ Adenosine is a purine nucleoside, used in ribonucleic and deoxyribonucleic acid biosynthesis.

---

* Second-degree AV block: not all impulses get through the AV node; third-degree AV block: no impulses get through the AV node.

† Sick sinus syndrome: a collection of abnormalities resulting in abnormally fast, irregular or slow impulse conduction through the AV node.

‡ Mainly associated with the low therapeutic index (margin of safety); digoxin has a very narrow margin between therapeutic and toxic effects.

* A neurotransmitter, binding to A1, A2 and A3 receptors in brain and heart.
* Uses:
  * anti-inflammatory, antiasthmatic, antidysrhythmic and possible anti-tumour agent; administration by rapid IV injection.
* Antidysrhythmic drug.
* Uses in arrhythmia:
  * treatment of choice for termination of paroxysmal supraventricular tachycardia, due to rapid onset and offset of action, i.e. low danger of adverse reactions
  * used diagnostically for complex supraventricular tachycardias.
* Adverse effects include:
  * bronchospasm
  * chest pain
  * dyspnoea (difficulty breathing) and sensation of choking
  * may be severe bradycardia.
* Precautions and contraindications:
  * arial flutter or fibrillation in patients with accessory conduction pathways in cardiac tissue
  * caution needed in heart transplant patients.
* Contraindications include:
  * patients with asthma
  * patients with 2nd or 3rd degree AV block
  * patients with sick sinus syndrome, except when fitted with a pacemaker.

Chapter 19 Quiz

ANSWER T (TRUE) F (FALSE)

1. Normal cardiac rhythm is:

   Controlled by the sino-atrial node and by autonomic inputs to the SA node. ☐

   Achieved through spread of electrical impulses through conducting tissues to atrial and ventricular muscles. ☐

2. Arrhythmias:

   Are deviations from normal sinus rhythm. ☐

   May be normal, temporary physiological responses. ☐

   Always occur continuously. ☐

   Produce symptoms of chest pain and 'palpitations'. ☐

   May in some cases be potentially life-threatening. ☐

3. Automaticity is caused by impulses from the S-A node. ☐

4. The aims of drug treatment are:

   To slow the heart and restore normal rhythm. ☐

   To correct abnormal pacemaker activity. ☐

5. Antidysrythmic drugs are classified according to:

   Their chemical structure. ☐

   Their site of action in the heart, e.g. supraventricular. ☐

   Their mechanism of action. ☐

6. Disopyramide and procainamide block fast Na^+ channels, which prolongs the duration of the action potential. ☐

7. They are usually reserved for supraventricular tachycardia. ☐

8. Lidocaine and mexiletine shorten action potential duration. ☐

9. They are used for life-threatening ventricular arrhythmias. ☐

10. Flecainide and propafenone lower rate of depolarisation of the AP* ☐

11. Lidocaine is used for emergencies, e.g. a heart attack. ☐

12. Lidocaine doses should be reduced after heart surgery or with CHF. ☐

13. Flecainide is used for:

    Treatment and prevention of paroxysmal atrial tachycardia. ☐

    Prevention of suspected life-threatening ventricular tachycardia. ☐

    Arrhythmias associated with Wolff-Parkinson-White syndrome. ☐

14. Flecainide is contraindicated in patients with a history of MI. ☐

15. Propranolol is a Class I antidysrhythmic drug. ☐

16. β-blockers are contradicted in patients with asthma. ☐

17. Amiodarone is a Class III antidysrhythmic drug. ☐

18. Amiodarone may cause thyroid dysfunction. ☐

19. Amiodarone is used to resuscitate during ventricular fibrillation. ☐

20. Verapamil is used to treat supraventricular tachycardias. ☐

21. Verapamil is contraindicated in patients with a history of heart failure. ☐

22. Verapamil is a K^+-channel blocker. ☐

23. Digoxin has a very narrow margin of safety. ☐

24. Digoxin slows the heart by suppressing vagal drive to it. ☐

25. Low plasma K^+ increases digoxin toxicity. ☐

26. Digoxin blood levels should be monitored during treatment. ☐

27. Adenosine is a pyrimidine nucleotide. ☐

28. Adenosine is the treatment of choice for terminating paroxysmal supraventricular tachycardia. ☐

* AP: action potential.

20 Drugs and the heart IV: angina pectoris

Learning objectives ■ Definition of angina pectoris ■ Symptoms ■ Stable and unstable angina ■ Risk factors for angina pectoris ■ Cause of angina pectoris ■ Triggers of anginal pain ■ Diagnosis of angina pectoris ■ Aims of treatment ■ Lifestyle changes ■ Drug treatment

---

Learning objectives

- Give a definition of angina pectoris.
- Be able to describe the symptoms.
- Know the difference between stable and unstable angina.
- Know the risk factors, causes and triggers for angina pectoris.
- Be aware of the diagnostic tools and aims of treatment.
- Know which lifestyle changes are recommended and the current drug treatments.

Definition of angina pectoris[*]

- Angina pectoris is chest pain caused by inadequate oxygen supply to cardiac tissues.

Symptoms

- Pain is often described as a crushing, severe pain and a sensation of suffocation and pressure just behind the breastbone (sternum); may be felt also in neck, arms and stomach.

Stable and unstable angina

- Stable angina is anginal pain due to atherosclerosis in coronary arteries.
- Unstable angina is most often due to plaque rupture and is usually signalled by new, sudden onset and severe anginal pain, usually lasting more than 15 minutes; either in cases of previously silent, undiagnosed, angina, or in patients previously with stable angina.

Note: unstable angina should be treated as an emergency as it may signal an imminent heart attack (myocardial infarction).

---

[*] Angina pectoris derivation: Greek – αγχειν *ankhein*: strangle or throttle; Latin – *pectoris*: of the chest.

Risk factors for angina pectoris

- Diabetes.
- Family history of angina pectoris.
- Hypercholesterolaemia.
- Hypertension.
- Sedentary lifestyle.
- Smoking.

Cause of angina pectoris

- Ischaemia (poor blood supply to the tissues), due mainly to spasm of coronary arteries or obstruction to blood flow (atherosclerosis) or both (*see* Figure 20.1).

Triggers of anginal pain

- Anything that speeds up the heart:
  - sudden or violent physical exertion
  - emotional stress
  - dreams
  - extremes of heat or cold weather
  - sometimes after meals.

Diagnosis of angina pectoris

- ECG during exercise on a treadmill (during anginal pain ST segment depression may be observed).
- Measurement of heart rate and rhythm during exercise.
- Thallium scintigram – areas of poor perfusion show up in X-rays as 'cold spots'.
- Coronary angiogram visualises flow though coronary arteries and reveals any occlusion or narrowing of arteries.

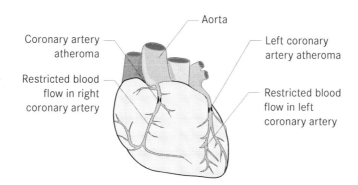

FIGURE 20.1 Atheromas in coronary arteries.

Aims of treatment

- Changes to lifestyle.
- Prevention of occurrence of pain.
- Treatment to ease anginal chest pain.
- Reduce rate of further atheroma deposition.
- Reduce the risk of myocardial infarction (heart attack).

Lifestyle changes

- Stop smoking.
- Limit alcohol intake to around 15–20 units of alcohol per week (men) and 14 units per week (women); men: not more than 4 units per day; women: not more than 3 units per day; 1 unit = 8 g of alcohol, e.g. 300 ml of 3.5% lager or beer or cider ; 125 ml wine.
- Weight reduction if overweight.
- Diet:
  - reduce fatty food intake; avoid fried food; stick to lean meat or poultry
  - increase intake of fruit and raw vegetables
  - eat oily fish, e.g. mackerel, herring, kippers
  - reduce salt intake.
- Do regular, gentle exercise to stimulate circulation through the heart; avoid sudden bursts of strenuous exercise.

Drug treatment

- Stable angina:
  - main aims of treatment:
    - symptomatic relief, i.e. ease the pain
    - reducing the rate of occurrence of painful episodes
    - slowing disease progression and reducing the chances of myocardial infarction and mortality.
- Symptomatic relief:
  - sublingual glyceryl trinitrate, a fast-acting vasodilator
  - longer acting nitrates, e.g. isosorbide dinitrate
  - dyhydropyridine-based calcium channel blockers, e.g. amlopidine (*see* safety note below)
  - ranolazine,[*] a newer piperazine derivative, which extends exercise time before anginal pain sets in.

Safety note: verapamil and diltiazem are contraindicated in patients with left ventricular dysfunction and are highly dangerous.

---

[*] Not listed in the BNF at the time of writing.

- Slowing disease progression:
  - low dose aspirin
  - β-blockers reduce both attack incidence and risk of mortality (but are contraindicated in patients with left ventricular dysfunction)
  - statins, e.g. atorvastatin, which inhibit cholesterol biosynthesis.
- Unstable angina:
  - on diagnosis, immediate admission to hospital as an emergency.
- Treat any underlying condition, e.g. fever or hypertension.
- Carry out blood tests and monitor ECG to test for and rule out myocardial infarction.
- Heparin infusion.
- Aspirin initially, perhaps replaced with clopidogrel for long-term therapy.
- Evidence of damaged cardiac tissue or significant ECG changes may require IIb/IIIa inhibitors, e.g. tirofiban or eptifibatide.
- Persistent symptoms of unstable angina may require Ca^{2+}-channel blockers or β-blockers, and cardiac catheterisation.
- Patients should be put onto long-term aspirin (75–300 mg) or clopidogrel.

Chapter 20 Quiz

ANSWER T (TRUE) F (FALSE)

1. Angina pectoris is chest pain caused by inadequate O_2 supply to heart muscle. ☐
2. Symptoms are crushing pain and suffocating chest sensations. ☐
3. Risk factors for angina pectoris include:

   Diabetes. ☐

   Family history of angina. ☐

   Hypercholesterolaemia. ☐

   A sedentary lifestyle. ☐

   Hypotension. ☐
4. Triggers for angina pectoris include:

   Sudden, sustained physical exertion. ☐

   Emotional stress. ☐

   Dreams. ☐

   After a meal. ☐
5. Unstable angina may herald an imminent heart attack. ☐

6. Diagnostic procedures for angina include:

   ECG. ☐

   Fasting glucose. ☐

   Monitoring heart rate and rhythm during exercise. ☐

   Thallium scintigram. ☐

   Coronary angiogram. ☐

7. Aims of treatment include:

   Prevent and stop the pain. ☐

   Reduce rate of atheroma deposition. ☐

   Reduce the risk of myocardial infarction. ☐

   Introduce lifestyle changes. ☐

   More strenuous exercise. ☐

8. Drug treatments include:

   Symptomatic relief with glyceryl trinitrate. ☐

   Use of longer-acting nitrates, e.g. isosorbide dinitrate. ☐

   Dyhydropyridine-based Ca^{2+}-channel blockers. ☐

   Statins to slow atheroma formation in coronary arteries. ☐

9. Unstable angina:

   When diagnosed requires immediate admission as an emergency. ☐

   Requires ECG monitoring. ☐

   May require heparin infusion and aspirin. ☐

   May require IIb/IIIa inhibitors, e.g. tirofiban or eptifibatide. ☐

   May require cardiac catheterisation. ☐

21 Drugs and the heart V: antiplatelet drugs

Learning objectives
- Know what blood platelets are.
- Be able to list some major activators of platelet aggregation.
- Know some serious consequences of platelet aggregation.
- Be able to list the currently used antiplatelet drugs and have some knowledge of their uses, mechanism of action and problems associated with their use.

Mini glossary
- Anaphylaxis: allergic reaction with widespread histamine release; can be fatal unless treated.
- Aneurism: balloon-like swelling in the arterial wall.
- Atherosclerosis: build-up of fatty deposits on endothelial walls of blood vessels.
- Canaliculi: small canals or channels.
- Haemostasis: physiological processes, namely coagulation and constriction of damaged blood vessels which arrest bleeding.
- Hapten: a small molecule that can combine with a body protein to form an antigen.
- Infarction: e.g. myocardial infarction (MI); death of local area of tissue due to interrupted blood supply.
- Ischaemic: having an inadequate blood flow to a tissue or organ caused by blood vessel blockage.
- Platelets: disc-shaped bodies in blood, 1.5–3 μm diameter, produced in bone marrow, involved in haemostasis.
- Reye's syndrome: relatively rare childhood syndrome of liver failure with symptoms of encephalitis linked to use of aspirin; aspirin should not be used in children under sixteen years.
- Thrombocytopaenia: blood platelet reduction.

Platelets

- Are disk-shaped, anuclear structures, 1.5–3 μm in diameter, in the blood of all mammals (*see* Figure 21.2).
- Are produced mainly in the bone marrow.
- Contain an outer membrane, contractile protein, RNA, a system of canaliculi, mitochondria and bodies containing several chemical mediators.
- Play a major role in the coagulation of blood.
- Are activated by:
  - epinephrine
  - adhesion to collagen, which is exposed when the blood vessel endothelium is damaged
  - contact with ADP, fibrinogen, thrombin and glass.
- Are activated through their surface receptors, which trigger:
  - thromboxane (Tx) production, e.g. TxA_2, which
  - activates platelet GPIIb/IIIa receptor, which
  - facilitates fibrinogen binding to platelets, which
  - results in platelet aggregation.
- When activated release inflammatory and other mediators, including:
  - platelet activator-4, which mediates arrest of monocytes on endothelium
  - nitric oxide
  - thrombospondin, which is involved in the process of platelet aggregation and atherosclerosis.
- When depleted in blood increase the chances of bleeding and haemorrhage.

TABLE 21.1 ACTIVATORS AND INHIBITORS OF PLATELET AGGREGATION

SOME NATURAL PLATELET ACTIVATORS	NATURAL PLATELET INHIBITORS	SYNTHETIC ANTI-PLATELET DRUGS
ADP	Adenosine	Abciximab
Collagen	Clotting factors II, IX, X, XI, XII	Aspirin
Epinephrine	Eptifibatide*	Clopidogrel
Human neutrophil elastase	Nitric oxide	NSAIDs
5-HT (serotonin)	Prostacyclin	Tirofiban**
Thrombin		
Thromboxane A_2		
Von Willebrand factor		

* Extract of snake venom (*see* text) marketed as Integrilin®
** Tirofiban (Aggrastat®)

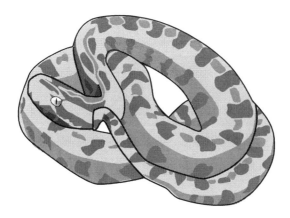

FIGURE 21.1 Pygmy rattlesnake (12–20 inches).

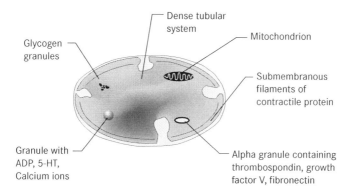

FIGURE 21.2 Structure of the platelet.

Antiplatelet drugs

- Aspirin.
- Abciximab.
- Eptifibatide.
- Tirofiban.

Aspirin

- In low doses blocks prostaglandin and therefore thromboxane TxA_2 synthesis by binding irreversibly to the COX-1 enzyme.
- In low doses is used to lower the risk of cardiovascular and cerebrovascular thrombus formation.
- Is given as soon as possible, preferably dispersed or chewable, after an ischaemic event in a larger (300 mg) dose and prescribed thereafter on a daily basis (75–300 mg daily).

117

- Is also prescribed for high risk patients in whom blood pressure is controlled for primary prevention of cardiovascular accidents.
- Adverse effects include:
  - inhibition of gastric mucus production, resulting in gastric bleeding
  - Reye's syndrome in young children (Do not give to children of 16 or under)
  - can be allergic as a hapten.

Clopidogrel

- Marketed by Plavix® Bristol-Myers Squibb/Sanofi-Synthelabo.
- Acts by blocking the binding of ADP to its platelet receptor (*see* Figure 21.3), thereby preventing ADP from activating the platelet GPIIb/IIIa receptor.
- Is taken orally in tablet form.
- Is used to protect patients with a history of atherosclerosis.
- Is useful for prevention of atherosclerotic events in peripheral arteries, if used within 35 days of myocardial infarction, or within 6 months after an ischaemic stroke.
- Is sometimes prescribed together with low dose aspirin, e.g. in acute coronary syndrome without ST-segment elevation*, although this combination increases bleeding risk.
- Should be started initially on hospital patients only.
- Should be used with caution in patients in whom there is any likelihood of bleeding, e.g. surgery.
- Adverse effects include:
  - GIT upsets, e.g. nausea, vomiting constipation, diarrhoea
  - thrombocytopaenia (relatively rare)
  - hypersensitivity reactions.

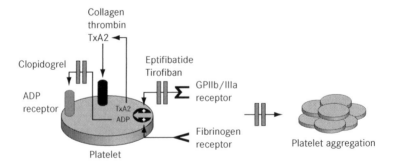

FIGURE 21.3 Mechanism of action of antiplatelet drugs.

---

* ST-segment elevation on the ECG may reflect, for example, impending infarction.

Abciximab

- Marketed by ReoPro® Lilly.
- Is a monoclonal antibody produced from the Fab fragments of an immunoglobulin designed to bind to the GPIIb/IIIa receptor.
- Binds to and blocks the GPIIb/IIIa receptor, which blocks platelet aggregation.
- Is used for patients undergoing percutaneous coronary surgery to prevent ischaemic cardiac complications.
- Is administered by IV injection or infusion.
- Use carries a risk of increased bleeding, especially if used with other drugs that increase bleeding risk.
- Should not be used when there is or has been:
  - active internal bleeding
  - trauma, intraspinal or intracranial surgery within the previous 2 months.[*]
- Adverse effects include:
  - bradycardia
  - hypersensitivity reactions
  - nausea
  - hypotension
  - back or chest pain
  - thrombocytopaenia.

Eptifibatide

- Marketed as Integrilin® GSK.
- Is a cyclic peptide extracted from the venom of a pygmy rattlesnake, *Sistrurus miliarus barbouri* (*see* Figure 21.1).
- Is used to prevent infarction in patients with:
  - early or non-ST-segment elevation myocardial infarction
  - with unstable angina
  - within the last episode of chest pain within 24 hours.
- Is administered by IV injection or infusion under specialist supervision.
- Is often administered together with:
  - aspirin or clopidogrel
  - heparin
  - nitrates, opioid analgesics
  - lidocaine (*see* pp. 101, 196).
- Adverse effects reported include:
  - anaphylaxis (rare)
  - bleeding; may be severe
  - cardiac arrhythmias and, relatively rarely, ventricular fibrillation
  - hypotension (low blood pressure)
  - thrombocytopaenia.

---

[*] *See* BNF for more details.

- Contraindications include:
  - intracranial diseases, e.g. aneurisms
  - major surgery
  - stroke within 30 days.

Tirofiban

- Marketed as Aggrastat® MSD.
- Is a synthetic, non-peptide GpIIb/IIIA receptor blocker.
- Inhibits platelet activation and aggregation.
- Is relatively fast-acting and of short duration.
- Is used for prevention of MI.
- Supplied as a sterile solution for IV infusion. (Cautionary note: it is also supplied as a concentrate for dilution; take care when dispensing; *see* BNF.)
- Is used together with aspirin and heparin as and when indicated.
- Is indicated for:
  - patients with non-ST-segment elevation MI*
  - unstable angina
  - if the last episode of chest pain occurred with 12 hours
  - before percutaneous transluminal coronary angioplasty
  - to reduce the incidence of refractory ischaemic states
  - to prevent a new MI.
- Adverse effects include:
  - bleeding, either at the site of application or elsewhere; rarely, bleeding may be severe
  - thrombocytopaenia, reversible, and observed more after concomitant heparin use
  - anaphylaxis (rare).
- Precautions with use include:
  - liver or kidney impairment
  - history of bleeding disorders, e.g. peptic ulcer, history of trauma or major surgery within 6 months
  - within two weeks of any tissue or organ biopsy
  - severe heart failure.
- Contraindications include:
  - any problems of increased prothrombin time
  - history of trauma or major surgery within 6 weeks
  - severe hypertension
  - intracranial problems including aneurisms
  - breast-feeding
  - any abnormal bleeding or stroke within 30 days.

---

* Non-ST-segment elevation MI: ST-segment elevation generally absent.

Chapter 21 Quiz

ANSWER T (TRUE) OR F (FALSE)

1. Platelets are used to widen arteries. ☐
2. Infarction is death of tissue through interrupted blood supply. ☐
3. Thrombocytopaenia is an excess of platelets. ☐
4. Platelets are activated by:

   Epinephrine. ☐

   Adhesion to collagen. ☐

   Contact with fibrinogen. ☐

   Contact with ADP. ☐

   Contact with thrombin. ☐

   Contact with glass. ☐
5. When activated inhibit thromboxane (TxA_2) synthesis. ☐
6. Platelets are biosynthesised mainly in bone marrow. ☐
7. Aspirin in low doses inhibits platelet activation by blocking TxA_2 synthesis. ☐
8. Aspirin is non-allergic. ☐
9. Clopidogrel inhibits platelet aggregation by enhancing ADP receptor activation. ☐
10. Abciximab inhibits platelet activation by blocking the GPIIb/IIIA receptor. ☐
11. Abciximab should not be used if there is a pre-existing bleeding risk. ☐
12. Eptifibatide is an anticoagulant factor derived from the venom of a snake. ☐
13. Tirofiban is a non-peptide antiplatelet drug given by IV infusion. ☐

22 Anticoagulants I: heparin, hirudins and heparinoids

Learning objectives ■ Coagulation of blood ■ Heparin ■ Low molecular weight heparins ■ Protamine sulphate – heparin antidote ■ Hirudins ■ Danaparoid sodium ■ Fondaparinux

Learning objectives

■ Know the difference between the extrinsic and intrinsic clotting systems.
■ Be able to list different drugs or drug types which target the coagulation cascade.
■ Know the nature, uses and dangers associated with heparin.
■ Be able to explain what low molecular weight heparins are, give some examples and list their advantages over heparin.
■ Know what hirudins and heparinoids are and be able to give examples.

Coagulation of blood

■ Is the conversion of blood from a liquid to a solid (*see* Figure 22.1).
■ Is primarily a device to arrest bleeding from a wound.
■ Is initiated by:
  ▮ contact with a foreign surface, e.g. air or glass (intrinsic system)
  ▮ a damaged tissue of the body (extrinsic system)
    ◆ the intrinsic pathway is activated when blood comes into contact with sub-endothelial connective tissues or with negatively charged surfaces exposed as a result of tissue damage
    ◆ the extrinsic pathway is an alternative route for the activation of the clotting cascade, providing a more rapid response to tissue injury, generating activated factor X almost instantaneously, compared to the seconds or even minutes taken by the intrinsic pathway to activate factor X. An important function of the extrinsic pathway is to augment the activity of the intrinsic pathway.
■ Involves the initiation of a cascade of reactions resulting ultimately in the formation of insoluble fibrin.
■ Results in the cessation of blood flow at the site of injury.
■ Is a target for several types of drugs including anticoagulants, to treat (for example):

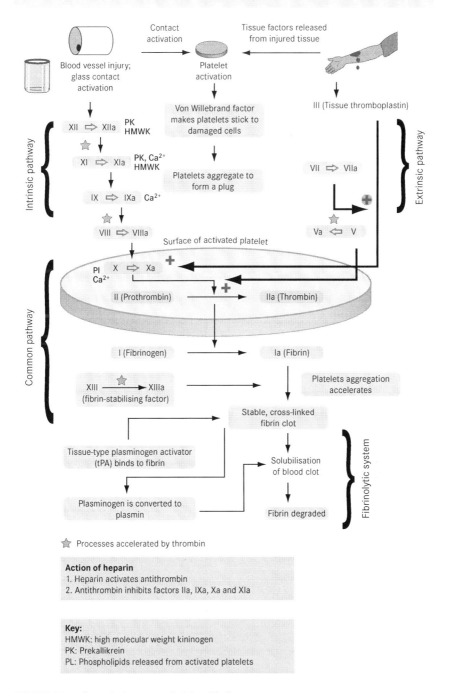

FIGURE 22.1 Coagulation cascade (simplifed).

- patients at high risk for in-stent* thrombosis after surgical procedures
- atrial fibrillation
- deep venous thrombosis
- pre-treatment before procedures such as angioplasty
- pulmonary embolism
- unstable angina.

Heparin

- Is a glycosaminoglycan.[†]
- Is a natural anticoagulant produced by basophils and mast cells.
- Acts by binding to antithrombin III (AT-III), which:
  - exposes the AT-III active site, which
  - inactivates thrombin and other protease enzymes, especially factor Xa
  - overall, potentiates AT-III activity x1000 (*see* Figure 22.1).
- Has a short biological half-life of ± 1 hour.
- Is inactivated by heparinase enzymes.
- Is used unfractionated for:
  - patients at high risk of bleeding because it has a short duration of action and can be stopped fast
  - prophylaxis in orthopaedic surgery
  - pulmonary embolism
  - rapid treatment of deep-venous thrombosis
  - management of myocardial infarction
  - management of unstable angina
  - management of acute peripheral arterial occlusion.
- Can be fractionated into low molecular weight heparins.
- Has adverse effects, including:
  - haemorrhage; a need to monitor aPTT[‡]
  - heparin-induced thrombocytopaenia
  - hypersensitivity reactions, including:
    - alopecia (hair loss; rare)
    - anaphylaxis
    - angioedema (oedema of deeper subcutaneous tissues caused by fluid leakage from dilated capillaries, resulting in large wheals)
    - urticaria
    - osteoporosis after prolonged use.
- Should be used with caution in:
  - patients with kidney or liver impairment

---

* Stent: device placed into a canal, for example a blood vessel, to maintain patency for liquid flow.
† Glycosaminoglycan: a polysaccharide with high molecular weight containing amino sugars; they often form complexes with proteins and are also referred to as mucopolysaccharides.
‡ aPTT: activated partial thromboplastin time; monitors rate of coagulation.

- elderly
- pregnancy
- patients who had hypersensitivity reactions to low molecular weight heparins.
- Is contraindicated:[*]
  - in acute bacterial endocarditis
  - after serious trauma or surgery to the eye or CNS
  - haemophilia or any other disorders involving haemorrhage
  - hypersensitivity to heparin
  - in thrombocytopaenia
  - any concomitant treatment, e.g. spinal anaesthesia when heparin is already part of the treatment.

Low molecular weight heparins
- Bemiparin.
- Dalteparin.
- Enoxaparin.
- Reviparin.
- Tinzaparin.
- Are prepared by fractionation and depolymerisation of native heparin.
- Different from unfractionated heparin in (for example):
  - molecular weight; heparin about 20 kDa;[†] low molecular weight heparins about 3 kDa
  - duration of action: dosage SC once daily vs. continuous IV infusion of heparin
  - perhaps a smaller bleeding risk; less need to monitor the aPTT
  - smaller risk of thrombocytopaenia
  - less risk of osteoporosis with long-term use
  - can be used on out-patients if appropriate
  - do not cross the placenta and may be used in pregnant patients under supervision
  - more suitable in hip and knee replacement surgery.
- Are usually administered by SC injection.
- Have similar adverse effects, precautions and contraindications as for unfractionated heparin.

Protamine sulphate – heparin antidote
- Is a highly basic peptide extracted from fish sperm.
- Binds to heparin and inactivates it.
- Is usually administered by IV injection.

---

[*] Patient status should always be thoroughly discussed before initiation of heparin treatment.
[†] kDa: kiloDaltons.

- Causes significant histamine release, with danger of hypotension, bradycardia and anaphylaxis.
- In higher doses has anticoagulant properties.

Hirudins

- Are anticoagulants derived from hirudin, found in the salivary glands of the medicinal leech *Hirudo medicinalis* (*see* Figure 22.2), now made using recombinant DNA technology; is called lepirudin.
- Bivalirudin is an hirudin analogue licensed for use in the UK.
- Mechanism of action is to bind to and inactivate the active form of thrombin.
- Are indicated as anticoagulants for patients who cannot take heparin due to, e.g. heparin-induced thrombocytopaenia.
- Are administered by IV injection and infusion.
- Are actually thrombolytic by dissolving the thrombus.
- Are contraindicated in:
  - patients with bleeding disorders
  - pregnant and breast-feeding patients (lepirudin)
  - patients with subacute bacterial endocarditis or severe hypertension.
- Should be used with caution in patients:
  - with liver or kidney impairment
  - who are pregnant or breast-feeding.*

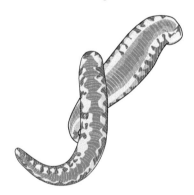

FIGURE 22.2 Medicinal leech *Hirudo medicinalis*.

Danaparoid sodium

- Is an example of a heparinoid, which are glycosaminoglycans derived from heparin.
- Is currently the only heparinoid listed in the BNF.

---

* *See* BNF for more details.

- Is a low molecular weight heparinoid which is derived from porcine gut mucosa.
- Contains as its active principles heparin, dermatan* and chondroitin as sulphates.
- Differs from low molecular weight heparins as it contains no heparin fragments.
- Acts (like heparin) mainly through inhibition of factor Xa.
- Is used to prevent deep venous thrombosis in (for example):
  - patients undergoing general or orthopaedic surgery
  - patients with a history of heparin-induced thrombocytopaenia.
- Should be used with caution in patients:
  - with kidney or liver impairment
  - where there is a risk of bleeding
  - in patients known to have antibodies to heparin
  - body weight over 90 kg (obesity has been linked with anti-factor Xa activity)
  - pregnancy and breast-feeding.
- Is contraindicated in patients with:
  - active peptic ulcer[†]
  - acute bacterial endocarditis
  - cerebral haemorrhage, if recent
  - haemophilia or other bleeding disorders
  - severe hypertension
  - thrombocytopaenia, except when caused by heparin
  - any treatment, e.g. spinal anaesthesia already containing danaparoid.
- Adverse effects include:
  - skin rashes
  - haemorrhage
  - hypersensitivity reactions.

Fondaparinux

- Is a synthetic pentasaccharide (a sugar).
- Is identical to the pentasaccharide sequence identified at the high affinity binding region for antithrombin-III.
- Acts by blocking the action of activated factor X.
- Has a significantly lower risk of thrombocytopaenia than heparin.
- Is contraindicated in patients with renal disease as fondaparinux is excreted via the kidneys.

---

* Dermatan is a mucopolysaccharide found mainly in skin; chondroitin is a glycosaminoglycan forming part of the ground substance of cartilage, bone and blood vessels.
† Unless peptic ulcer is the reason for operating.

Chapter 22 Quiz

ANSWER T (TRUE) OR F (FALSE)

1. Coagulation is the conversion of liquid to solid blood. ☐
2. Is initiated by tissue damage or blood contact with, e.g. glass. ☐
3. Coagulation is a target for drugs that treat (for example):

   Atrial fibrillation. ☐

   Deep venous thrombosis. ☐

   Pulmonary embolism. ☐

   Stable angina. ☐

4. Heparin:

   Is chemically a glycosaminoglycan. ☐

   Is produced by basophils and mast cells. ☐

   Inactivates thrombin and factor Xa. ☐

   Potentiates antithrombin (AT-III) activity 1000-fold. ☐

   Is inactivated by heparinase enzymes. ☐

   Has a long half-life. ☐

   Carries a serious risk of thrombocytopaenia. ☐

   Carries a risk of osteoporosis with long-term use. ☐

5. Heparin is used for:

   Prophylaxis in orthopaedic surgery. ☐

   Thrombocytopaenia. ☐

   Pulmonary embolism. ☐

   Management of myocardial infarction. ☐

   Management of acute peripheral arterial occlusion. ☐

   Procedures that require a quickly reversible anticoagulant. ☐

   Rapid treatment of deep venous thrombosis. ☐

6. LMWH* need more frequent dosage than unfractionated heparin. ☐
7. LMWH are prepared by fractionating native heparin. ☐
8. LMWH need be given once daily only by SC injection. ☐
9. LMWH usually carry a greater bleeding risk than does heparin. ☐
10. LMWH:

    Include bemiparin, dalteparin, enoxaparin, reviparin, tinzaparin. ☐

    Carry a smaller risk of thrombocytopaenia than does heparin. ☐

    Carry a lesser risk of osteoporosis with long-term use. ☐

    Can be used with out-patients. ☐

11. LMWH have generally similar precautions for use as heparin. ☐
12. Hirudins are anticoagulants derived from the skin of a frog. ☐
13. Lepirudin is recombinant hirudin. ☐
14. Hirudins bind to and inactivate the active form of thrombin. ☐
15. Hirudins are used for patients who cannot take heparin. ☐
16. Hirudins also lyse the blot clot. ☐
17. Hirudins are contraindicated in pregnancy. ☐
18. Hirudins require caution in patients with liver or kidney problems. ☐
19. Danaparoid sodium is a heparinoid derived from heparin. ☐
20. Fondaparinux is an anticoagulant that inactivates activated factor X. ☐
21. Protamine sulphate is an antidote for heparin. ☐

* LMH: low molecular weight heparins.

23 Anticoagulants II: oral anticoagulants

Learning objectives ■ Oral anticoagulants ■ Vitamin K ■ Warfarin sodium ■ Clinical use of warfarin ■ Drug interactions with warfarin ■ Adverse effects of warfarin ■ Precautions with warfarin ■ Contraindications with warfarin ■ Other oral anticoagulants ■ Acenocoumarol ■ Phenindione

Learning objectives

- Know the names of the three main oral anticoagulants in use.
- Know the mechanism of action of the oral anticoagulants on vitamin K.
- Be able to list the main clinical indications for the use of the oral anticoagulants.
- Be aware of the implications of hepatic enzyme induction and warfarin action.
- Be able to explain why the onset action of warfarin is delayed.
- Know which class of coagulation factors are affected by warfarin and how.
- Be aware of the importance of drug interactions with warfarin and be able to give some examples and consequences of the interactions.
- Know the chief dangers attached to the use of warfarin.
- Be able to list some important adverse effects, precautions and contraindications with warfarin.
- Be especially aware of the dangers of warfarin use in pregnancy.

Oral anticoagulants

- Include warfarin, acenocoumarol, phenindione.
- Are a group of anticoagulants that can be taken orally.
- Can be taken at home under medical supervision.
- Act by antagonising the effects of vitamin K.
- Have a delayed onset of action (48–72 hours).
- Are indicated mainly for:
  - deep-vein thrombosis
  - atrial fibrillation with risk of embolisation*
  - pulmonary embolism

---

* Embolisation is a block to blood flow caused by, for example, a blood clot.

- patients with prosthetic mechanical heart valves
- after diagnosis of a transient ischaemic attack.
- Are associated with significant bleeding risk with overdose, therefore require close patient monitoring and patient compliance to reduce the risk of overdose.
- Warfarin is associated with extensive drug interactions.

Vitamin K

- Is a fat-soluble vitamin synthesised by bacteria in the large intestine; occurs also in green plants.
- Is a cofactor required for the carboxylase enzyme that generates the production of gammacarboxyglutamic acid residues on (for example):
  - coagulation factors II, VII, IX and X (the vitamin K-dependant coagulation factors; *see* Figure 23.1)
  - protein S, protein C and protein Z, which are components of the coagulation process.
- Goes through a cycle of oxidation and reduction which regenerates fresh vitamin K.
- Can be blocked by oral anticoagulants, e.g. warfarin, which block the reduction of vitamin K oxide to vitamin K.

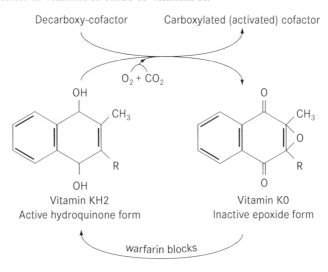

FIGURE 23.1 Actions of vitamin K and warfarin.

Warfarin sodium

- Is an oral anticoagulant.
- Is a coumarin derivative.
- Is a racemic mixture of two optically active isomers R- and S-warfarin,

S-warfarin being the more potent isomer with respect to anti-vitamin K action.

- Was originally discovered through the death by haemorrhage of cattle by spoiled sweet clover in the USA and Canada.
- Was originally introduced as a rat poison.[*]
- Is taken orally in tablet form.
- Has a delay in onset dictated by the half-lives of the vitamin-K dependent clotting factors (the shortest being VII, with a half-life of 3–4 hours).
- Is associated with a large number of drug interactions.

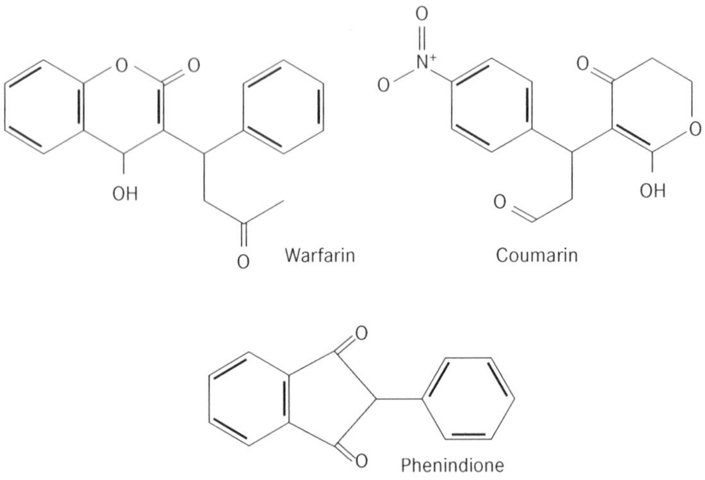

Warfarin   Coumarin

Phenindione

FIGURE 23.2 Structures of oral anticoagulants (compare with Vitamin K).

Clinical use of warfarin

- The baseline prothrombin time, reported as the INR,[†] should be measured but warfarin started before the result is obtained.
- Warfarin is supplied in tablet form for oral use.
- Prescribed initially as a single loading dose followed by a lower maintenance dose depending on the patient's INR and condition.
- INR should be monitored, preferably daily during early treatment stages, then regularly thereafter; accidental overdose, changes in the patient's clinical status and patient compliance have to be taken into account.
- In case of raised INR, depending on INR value:
  - stop warfarin until acceptable INR is obtained and restart warfarin
  - in case of haemorrhage, stop warfarin and administer:

---

[*] Some believe warfarin was used to poison Stalin.
[†] INR: International Normalized Ratio; see BNF for more details.

+ phytomenadione (vitamin K_1)*
+ prothrombin complex (a mixture of factors II, VII, IX and X) or fresh frozen plasma.

Drug interactions with warfarin

(*Note*: this is not a comprehensive list.)[†]

* Drugs that potentiate warfarin action:
  * inhibitors of liver microsomal metabolising enzymes:
    + antibiotics, e.g. chloramphenicol, ciprofloxacin
    + H_2-receptor blockers, e.g. cimetidine
    + antidepressants, e.g. imipramine
    + antidysrhythmic drugs, e.g. amiodarone.
  * inhibitors of platelet function, e.g. NSAIDs such as aspirin.
  * drugs that interfere with vitamin K availability (for example):
    + cephalosporins, which inhibit vitamin K reduction
    + antibiotics which destroy normal GIT flora, e.g. broad spectrum antibiotics.

Dietary warning note: cranberry juice contains antioxidant flavonoids which inhibit liver microsomal P450 enzymes, thus potentiating warfarin action. At least one fatality has occurred with cranberry juice and warfarin.

* Drugs that reduce warfarin potency by inducing microsomal enzymes:
  * barbiturates
  * oral contraceptives
  * anti-epileptics, e.g. phenytoin.

Adverse effects of warfarin[‡]

* Haemorrhage.
* Hypersensitivity reactions.
* Nausea and vomiting.
* Jaundice.
* Fall in haematocrit.[§]
* Diarrhoea.
* Alopecia (scalp hair loss).
* Pancreatitis.
* Liver disorders.

---

* Vitamin K_1 is methyl-3-(3,7,11,15-tetramethylhexadec-2-enyl) naphthalene-1,4-dione; found in green plants; also called phytomenadione.
† The list of drugs is actually enormous and warfarin prescribers must do a thorough and on-going check of other medications being taken when putting patients onto warfarin.
‡ Warfarin accounts for about 15% of all reported drug-related adverse effects in the UK.
§ Haematocrit: ratio of packed red cell volume/whole blood volume.

- Osteoporosis reported after prolonged use.
- Skin rashes, skin necrosis at site of injection.
- Thrombocytopaenia may occur after 6–10 days of warfarin; platelet counts should be done 5 days after initiation of warfarin therapy.

Precautions with warfarin

- Impaired liver or kidney function.
- Pregnancy and breast-feeding.
- Third trimester and delivery bleeding risk; warfarin should be avoided.*
- Warfarin does not appear to enter breast milk but should be used with caution during breast-feeding and it may be prudent to monitor the baby's prothrombin time.

Teratogenicity note: the greatest risk to the foetus with warfarin is weeks 6–9 of gestation. Warfarin must not be used in the first trimester of pregnancy, and ideally should not be used in the third trimester either, unless unavoidable.

Contraindications with warfarin

- Alcoholism (damaged liver).
- Any bleeding disorder, e.g. peptic ulcer.
- Bacterial endocarditis.
- Pregnancy, especially first and third trimesters (*see* above).
- Recent CNS surgery.
- Severe hypertension.

Other oral anticoagulants

- Acenocoumarol.
- Phenindione.

Acenocoumarol

- Also known as Nicoumalone, marketed as Sinthrome® Alliance.
- A derivative of coumarin (the natural anticoagulant found in plants).
- Indications, adverse effects, precautions and contraindications as for warfarin.
- Avoid during pregnancy and while breast-feeding.

Phenindione

- Properties and uses are similar to those of the other oral anticoagulants.
- Relatively rarely used; prescribed if patients experience idiosyncratic anti-warfarin reactions.

---

* The physician faces a difficult decision shortly before or at delivery if the mother has atrial fibrillation, pulmonary embolism, a history of venous thrombosis or a prosthetic heart valve.

Chapter 23 Quiz

ANSWER T (TRUE) OR F (FALSE)

1. Oral anticoagulants are taken by mouth. ☐
2. Have a delayed onset of action. ☐
3. Warfarin:
    Blocks active vitamin K biosynthesis. ☐
    Can be taken by the patient at home. ☐
    Is associated with extensive drug interactions. ☐
    Is a fat-soluble vitamin. ☐
4. Warfarin action is potentiated by:
    Inhibitors of liver microsomal enzymes. ☐
    Some antibiotics, e.g. ciprofloxaxin. ☐
    Vitamin K. ☐
    Antidepressants, e.g. imipramine. ☐
    H2-receptor blockers, e.g. cimetidine. ☐
    Cephalosporins, which inhibit vitamin K reduction. ☐
    Inhibitors of platelet function, e.g. aspirin. ☐
5. Adverse effects of warfarin include:
    Haemorrhage. ☐
    Fall in haematocrit. ☐
    Liver disorders. ☐
    Pancreatitis. ☐
    Osteoporosis with prolonged use. ☐
    Thrombocytopaenia. ☐
    Hypersensitivity reactions. ☐
6. Contraindications with warfarin include:
    Alcoholism. ☐
    Severe hypertension. ☐
    First and third trimesters of pregnancy. ☐
    Recent CNS surgery. ☐
    Bacterial endocarditis. ☐
    Bleeding disorders, e.g. peptic ulcer. ☐
7. Precautions with warfarin include:
    Breast-feeding. ☐
    Pregnancy. ☐
    Impaired pituitary function. ☐

24 Fibrinolytic and antifibrinolytic drugs

Learning objectives ■ Fibrinolysis ■ Plasmin ■ Antifibrinolytic drugs ■ Aprotinin ■ Tranexamic acid ■ Fibrinolytic drugs

Learning objectives

- Know what is meant by fibrinolysis.
- Be able to explain briefly the actions of plasmin.
- Know briefly what plasmin and tranexamic acid are, how they act and are used.
- Be able to explain the basic differences between first, second and third generation fibrinolytic drugs, how they act and their uses.

Fibrinolysis

- Is digestion of fibrin by the enzyme plasmin, thus dissolving a blood clot (*see* Figure 24.1).
- Ensures the removal of the blood clot from the circulation, thus ensuring a healthy balance between normal coagulation and fibrinolysis.
- Depends on the action of the proteolytic enzyme plasmin.

Plasmin

- Is a proteolytic enzyme formed from plasminogen (*see* Figure 24.1).
- Is produced by plasminogen activators:
  - tissue-type plasminogen activator (tPA)
  - urokokinase-type plasminogen activator (uPA)
  - kallikrein
  - neutrophil elastase.
- Targets specifically lysine and arginine residues at the C-terminal.
- Digests insoluble fibrin to release soluble fibrin degradation products (FDPs).*
- Potentiates its own activity by promoting tPA and uPA production.
- Activity is terminated mainly by α_2-antiplasmin (plasmin inhibitor) and $\alpha2$-macroglobulin.

---

* FDPS can be measured in blood and are used as markers of fibrinolysis in pulmonary embolism and deep vein thrombosis.

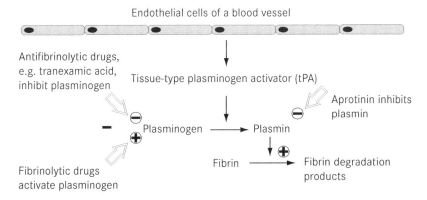

FIGURE 24.1 The fibrinolytic system and fibrinolyic and antifibrinolytic drug action.

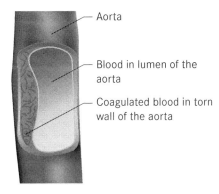

FIGURE 24.2 Aortic dissection.

Antifibrinolytic drugs

- Include:
  - aprotinin
  - tranexamic acid.
- Are drugs that inhibit fibrinolysis.
- Are used to prevent bleeding in (for example):
  - dentistry with haemophiliac patients
  - epistaxis (nosebleed)
  - hereditary angio-oedema*
  - surgery
  - menorrhagia (abnormally heavy menstrual bleeding)
  - prostatectomy
  - overdosage with thrombolytic drugs
  - transplantation procedures.

---

* Oedema involving eyes, lips and tongue.

Aprotinin
- Is a protein also known as bovine pancreatic trypsin inhibitor.
- Is licensed for use in the UK to reduce bleeding during open heart surgery and for hyperplasminaemia.
- Is a serine protease inhibitor, blocking mainly:
  - chymotrypsin
  - plasmin
  - kallikrein
  - trypsin.
- Is administered as IV injection or infusion.
- Adverse effects reported include:
  - anaphylaxis
  - thrombophlebitis.
- Precautions include pregnancy and breast-feeding.
- Contraindications include use in children.

Tranexamic acid
- Is a synthetic drug which competitively inhibits conversion of plasminogen to plasmin.
- Is used to treat:
  - menorrhagia
  - angioedema
  - haemophilia in dentistry
  - in cardiac surgery.
- Is administered as oral tablets and as an IV injection.
- Adverse effects reported include:
  - colour vision disturbance (discontinue the drug)
  - diarrhoea (when dose should be reduced).
- Should be used with caution in:
  - pregnancy
  - kidney disease
  - haematuria (presence of blood in urine).
- Is contraindicated in:
  - severe kidney disease
  - thromboembolic disease.

Fibrinolytic drugs
- Activate plasminogen to form plasmin which degrades the fibrin blood clot.
- Reduce mortality in patients suffering from myocardial infarction.
- Can be classified as:[*]
  - first generation, e.g. streptokinase, urokinase
  - second generation, e.g. alteplase
  - third generation, e.g. reteplase, tenecteplase.

---

[*] Not comprehensive; many more 3rd generation fibrinolytics are in development.

FIRST GENERATION FIBRINOLYTIC DRUGS

- Streptokinase:
  - is an enzyme produced by β-haemolytic streptococcus
  - binds to plasminogen and converts it to plasmin
  - is indicated for life-threatening cases (for example):
    - acute arterial thromboembolism
    - acute myocardial infarction
    - central retinal thrombosis
    - deep vein thrombosis (DVT)
    - pulmonary embolism
    - is administered by IV injection or infusion
    - is not specific for clot-bound fibrin but circulating fibrin as well, causing loss of circulating fibrin, which increases the bleeding risk
    - is antigenic – patients may develop antibodies to streptokinase.
- Urokinase:
  - is a serine protease originally isolated from human urine, but can be isolated from kidney parenchymal* cell cultures
  - is licensed for use to:
    - free cannulae and intravascular cannulae which become blocked with fibrin clots
    - treat DVT
    - treat peripheral vascular occlusion
    - treat pulmonary embolism.
  - is associated with concerns about inadvertent transmission of disease if derived from human source material.

SECOND GENERATION FIBRINOLYTIC DRUGS

- Alteplase:
  - is a recombinant human tissue type plasminogen activator, also known as rt-PA)
  - was originally cloned from a human melanoma cell line
  - has very high affinity for fibrin
  - the alteplase-fibrin complex formed then binds plasminogen at the clot and converts the plasminogen to plasmin, producing *local* fibrinolysis selectively
  - is indicated for:
    - acute ischaemic stroke
    - acute myocardial infarction

---

* Parenchymal: describes the functional tissues of an organ as opposed to the supporting tissue (stroma).

- ♦ pulmonary embolism
- ♦ has been used also to free occluded catheters
- is administered by IV injection and infusion.

THIRD GENERATION FIBRINOLYTIC DRUGS

- Were developed to produce drugs more specific for clot-bound fibrin.
- To improve safety and efficacy.
- To prolong duration of action, i.e. to extend the drugs half-life.
- Reteplase:
  - is a modified recombinant non-glycosylated[*] human tissue plasminogen
  - binds fibrin with a lower affinity than does alteplase; therefore it can penetrate deeper into the clot
  - administration by IV infusion.
- Tenecteplase:
  - targets fibrin with higher specificity than does alteplase
  - is more resistant than alteplase to PAI-1[†]
  - is a genetically modified form of tissue plasminogen activator
  - has a longer half-life than has alteplase and can therefore be given as a single IV dose rather than as an infusion.[‡]
- Adverse effects of the fibrinolytic agents include:
  - bleeding, usually at the injection site, but may occur at other sites, including intracranial
  - hypersensitivity reactions
  - hypotension
  - nausea and vomiting.
- Precautions with fibrinolytic drugs include:
  - hypertension
  - ongoing or recently discontinued anticoagulant therapy
  - any invasive procedure
  - any pre-existing condition when there is a risk that thrombolysis might precipitate bleeding
  - pregnancy
  - menstruation.
- Contraindications to the use of fibrinolytic agents:[§]
  - any history of a cerebral haemorrhage
  - any cerebral vascular incident within the last 12 months
  - any recent surgery, including dental surgery
  - any identified cranial neoplasm

---

[*] Glycosylated: addition of glycosyl groups to a protein to produce a glycoprotein.
[†] PAI-1 is plasminogen activator inhibitor-1 and it inhibits plasminogen activator.
[‡] *See* BNF for more details.
[§] Not comprehensive.

▌ any internal bleeding

▌ known or suspected aortic dissection* (*see* Figure 24.2).

Chapter 24 Quiz

ANSWER T (TRUE) OR F (FALSE)

1. Fibrinolysis is digestion of fibrin. ☐
2. Plasmin is a proteolytic enzyme formed from plasminogen. ☐
3. Plasmin is produced from kallikrein. ☐
4. Plasmin cuts specifically arginine and lysine C-terminal junctions. ☐
5. Antifibrinolytic drugs inhibit fibrinolysis. ☐
6. Antifibrinolytic drugs are used to promote bleeding. ☐
7. Antifibrinolytics help to control bleeding during surgery. ☐
8. Aprotinin is a serine protease inhibitor. ☐
9. Aprotinin is administered mainly by IV infusion or injection. ☐
10. Tranexamic acid is extracted from platelets. ☐
11. Tranexamic acid inhibits conversion of plasminogen to plasmin. ☐
12. Tranexamic acid cannot be administered orally. ☐
13. Fibrinolytic drugs promote breakdown of the fibrin clot. ☐
14. Fibrinolytic drugs activate plasminogen to form plasmin. ☐
15. Streptokinase is a first generation fibrinolytic drug. ☐
16. Streptokinase is currently indicated mainly for life-threatening cases. ☐
17. Streptokinase converts plasmin to plasminogen. ☐
18. Streptokinase is an enzyme derived from streptococcus. ☐
19. Streptokinase is used in acute myocardial infarction. ☐
20. Alteplase is also known as rt-PA. ☐
21. Alteplase binds to fibrin. ☐
22. The alteplase-fibrin complex converts plasminogen to plasmin. ☐
23. Third generation fibrinolytics are more specific for clot-bound fibrin. ☐

---

* Aortic dissection: bleeding into arterial wall through a tear in the endothelial lining – potentially life-threatening (*see* Figure 24.2).

25 Hypertension I: introduction

Learning objectives
- Know the difference between systolic and diastolic blood pressure.
- Know how blood pressure is expressed.
- Be able to list the main physiological factors that determine blood pressure.
- Be aware of the difference between primary and secondary hypertension.
- Know what is meant by primary (essential) and secondary hypertension.
- Be ready to list some consequences and risks associated with persistent hypertension.
- Be able to list some important diagnostic tests for diagnosis of hypertension.

Blood pressure parameters
- Systolic blood pressure: arterial pressure due to heart contractions.
- Diastolic blood pressure: arterial pressure when heart is not contracting; is due to resistance offered to flow by (mainly) arterial vessels.

Expression of parameters
- Expressed as systolic/diastolic pressure in mmHg,[*] e.g. 120/80, where 120 = systolic pressure; 80 = diastolic pressure.

Normal control of blood pressure
- Main physiological factors that determine blood pressure:[†]
    - rate and force of cardiac contraction
    - activity of the renin-angiotensin-aldosterone system
    - resistance to blood flow offered by the peripheral blood vessels
    - the baroreceptor reflex.

---

[*] Hg: mercury.
[†] Although listed separately, all the factors listed are interdependent in the determination of blood pressure.

Parameter note: systolic pressure may be raised normally due to, e.g. exercise, stress etc, and does not necessarily signal disease. Consistent abnormally raised diastolic pressure reflects raised resistance to flow and is more likely to reflect a possible underlying disease cause.

A definition of hypertension

- Hypertension is consistently measured blood pressure of 140/90 mmHg or more; patients may or may not need treatment depending on risk evaluation; blood pressure of 160/90–100 consistently, flags definite clinical hypertension.

Classification of hypertension

- Essential hypertension – the most frequent; cause unknown but linked to narrowing of arterial vessels through atheroma.
- Secondary hypertension – caused as a symptom of, e.g. endocrine disease, particularly related to adrenal function, which unbalances salt and water metabolism, kidney disease or phaeochromocytoma (*see* below).

Consequences and increased risks with persistent hypertension

- Hypertensive cardiomyopathy – hypertension associated with diseased heart muscle.
- Increased risk of myocardial infarction (heart attack).
- Increased risk of stroke.
- Hypertensive retinopathy – damage to the retinal blood vessels and possible blindness caused by retinal vessel rupture due to high blood pressure.
- Hypertensive nephropathy – renal damage and failure due to high perfusion pressure because of high blood pressure.

Diagnosis of hypertension

- Measurement of blood pressure.
- Distinction between essential hypertension (unknown aetiology) and secondary hypertension, which is secondary to, e.g. catecholamine-secreting tumours (phaeochromocytoma), using:
  - blood tests for catecholamines
  - measurement of electrolytes, especially, K^+ and Na^+
  - measurement of blood glucose (for diabetes)
  - check for kidney damage by measuring creatinine and urine proteins.

Chapter 25 Quiz

ANSWER T (TRUE) OR F (FALSE)

1. Systolic pressure is due to heart contraction. ☐
2. Diastolic pressure is due to the arterial resistance to blood flow. ☐
3. Blood pressure is expressed in mmHg (mercury). ☐
4. Blood pressure is normally controlled by:
   Rate and force of cardiac contraction. ☐
   Activity of the RAAS* system. ☐
   Resistance offered by the peripheral blood vessels. ☐
   The baroreceptor reflex. ☐
   Diet. ☐
5. Abnormally high diastolic pressure may reflect hypertension.
6. Persistently raised BP (e.g. 140/90 mmHg) reflects hypertension.
7. Possible consequences of persistent hypertension include:
   Hypertensive cardiomyopathy. ☐
   Increased risk of myocardial infarction. ☐
   Hypertensive retinopathy. ☐
   Hypertensive nephropathy. ☐
   Syncope (fainting). ☐
8. Diagnostic tools for hypertension include:
   Measurement of blood pressure. ☐
   Blood tests for abnormally high catecholamines.† ☐
   Measurement of plasma K^+, Na^+ and creatinine.‡ ☐
   Measurement of blood glucose (test for diabetes). ☐

* Renin-angiotensin-aldosterone system.
† To distinguish essential from secondary hypertension.
‡ Check for kidney damage.

26 Hypertension II: treatment

Learning objectives ■ Treatment of hypertension ■ Treatment strategy summarised ■ Lifestyle and dietary counselling ■ Treatment with drugs ■ Use of drugs ■ Drug treatment strategies ■ Individual drug classes ■ Direct vasodilators

Learning objectives

- Know examples of all the main classes of drugs used for hypertension with some precautions and contraindications in each group.
- Be able to give a brief account of lifestyle and dietary recommendations.

Treatment of hypertension[*]

- Changes in lifestyle:
  - diet
  - exercise.
- Drugs:
  - ACE inhibitors
  - angiotensin-II receptor blockers (ARBs)
  - β-blockers
  - α-blockers
  - calcium channel blockers
  - diuretics
  - direct vasodilators
  - direct renin inhibitor (Aliskerin).[†]

Treatment strategy summarised[‡]

- Treatment thresholds:
  - blood pressure: systolic 140–159 mmHg or diastolic 90–99 mmHg: + no organ damage + no cardiovascular complications:
    - ◆ treatment: lifestyle and dietary counselling; no drugs; monthly check-ups
  - blood pressure: systolic 140–159 mmHg or diastolic 90–99 mmHg + evidence of organ damage or cardiovascular complications or diabetes:
    - ◆ treatment: lifestyle and dietary counselling + drug therapy if patient's condition and raised BP values are sustained for 12 weeks

---

[*] Essential hypertension: hypertension of unknown aetiology.
[†] Aliskerin (Rasilez® Novartis); not yet available in the UK at the time of writing.
[‡] Based on BNF recommendations March 2007.

- blood pressure: systolic 160–179 mmHg or diastolic 100–109 mmHg + no organ damage + no cardiovascular complications:
  - treatment: lifestyle and dietary counselling; monitor weekly + drug therapy if patient's condition and raised BP values are sustained over 4–12 weeks
- blood pressure: systolic 160–179 mmHg or diastolic 100–109 mmHg + cardiovascular complications + organ damage or diabetes with symptoms persisting over 3–4 weeks:
  - treatment: lifestyle and dietary counselling; monitor + drug therapy if patient's condition and raised BP values are sustained over 3–4 weeks
- blood pressure: systolic 180–219 mmHg or diastolic 110–119 mmHg:
  - treatment: lifestyle and dietary counselling; monitor + drug therapy if patient's condition and raised BP values are sustained over 1–2 weeks
- blood pressure: systolic ≥ 220 mmHg or diastolic ≥129 mmHg:
  - treatment: lifestyle and dietary counselling + treat immediately with drugs.

Lifestyle and dietary counselling

- Reduce weight if appropriate.
- Exercise.
- Avoid fatty 'fast foods' and increase vegetable and fruit intake.
- Stop smoking[*] and reduce alcohol intake.
- Reduce salt intake.
- Increase calcium intake.

Treatment with drugs

- Aim of treatment:
  - for most patients, aim to keep blood pressure below 140/90
  - for patients with diabetes or renal disease, some recommend keeping BP below 120/80.

Use of drugs[†]

- Classes of drugs used:
  - thiazide diuretics, e.g. bendroflumethiazide
  - β-blockers, e.g. atenolol
  - α-blockers, e.g. prazocin

---

[*] This is to reduce dangers of heart attacks and stroke associated with long-term hypertension and with bad diet and smoking.
[†] A fluid area of recommendation, with some consensus; no doubt some ideas will have changed by the time you read this.

- calcium channel blockers, e.g. diltiazem
- ACE inhibitors, e.g. captopril
- angiotensin-II receptor antagonists, e.g. losartan
- drugs acting centrally, e.g. clonidine
- direct renin inhibitors, e.g. aliskiren.*

Drug treatment strategies *(see Figure 26.1)*[†]

- Younger white patients (under 55): ACE inhibitors preferred initially over thiazides and Ca^{2+}-channel blockers.
- Black patients do not generally respond well to initial use of ACE inhibitors.
- Patients 55 or older: thiazides or Ca^{2+}-channel blockers may be most likely to be effective.
- β-blockers not currently considered suitable as initial therapy for uncomplicated hypertension.
- Ca^{2+}-channel blockers differ in indications for use:
  - diltiazem and verapamil are favoured in patients with angina
  - dyhydropyridine-based Ca^{2+}-channel blockers, e.g. amlodipine, are recommended for elderly patients with isolated systolic hypertension, who cannot tolerate thiazides
  - α-blockers have adverse effects, e.g. postural hypotension, and are used in combination when hypertension is resistant to other treatments.
- Combining drug treatments: a two-pronged attack on high blood pressure might consist of ACE inhibitor + calcium channel blocker, or a diuretic.
- Angiotensin- II receptor blockers may be used for patients who cannot tolerate ACE inhibitors.
- Aim for longer-acting drugs with fewer longer between-dose intervals, taking into account the individual patient's health status and compliance.
- Inform patients fully about the choices and known adverse effects before prescribing drugs.

INDIVIDUAL DRUG CLASSES
DIURETICS
Examples: thiazides and thiazide-related compounds
- Bendroflumethiazide.
- Chlortalidone.
- Cyclopenthiazide.

---

* Aliskiren: a new treatment at time of writing.
† Patient requirements may vary; not comprehensive.

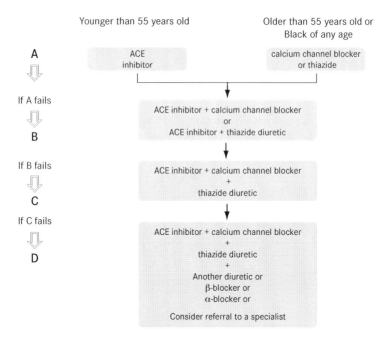

Adapted from: National Institute for Health and Clinical Excellence, June 2006. Hypertension: management of hypertension in adults in primary care.

FIGURE 26.1 Prescribing guide for new patients diagnosed with hypertension.

Mechanism of action
- Inhibition of Na^+ and Cl^- reabsorption in the distal tubule of the kidney.
- Vasodilation through desensitising smooth muscle to norepinephrine-induced intracellular Ca^{2+} release.

Uses
- Often the first-line drugs in newly-diagnosed hypertension.
- Prevention of formation of renal calculi (kidney stones) by reducing Ca^{2+} excretion in the kidney.
- In combination with ACE inhibitors (*see* p. 153) to reduce K^+ loss and in more severe cases of hypertension.
- Available in oral table form.

Adverse effects*
- Potassium loss (dangerous in patients with coronary artery disease).
- Gastrointestinal upsets.
- Hyperglycaemia.

---

* Not comprehensive; *see* BNF for more details.

- Hyperuricaemia.
- Impotence.
- Altered plasma lipids.

Precautions and contraindications
- Use lower doses initially in elderly patients.
- Use with caution in patients with gout, kidney or liver disease, SLE,* and in pregnant or breast-feeding woman.
- Do not use in patients with Addison's disease (adrenal insufficiency), electrolyte imbalances including hypercalcaemia and hyponatraemia (low blood Na^+), or patients on digoxin, which is made more toxic with lowered blood potassium.

β-BLOCKERS
Examples[†]
- Propranolol – the first introduced; binds both β_1-and β_2-adrenoceptors.
- Atenolol, esmolol; β_1-selective.

Mechanisms of action
- β_1-receptors on cardiac muscle increase rate and force of contraction; thus β_1-blockers slow the heart.
- β_2-receptors on arteriolar blood vessel walls dilate vessels, thus reducing peripheral resistance to blood flow.

Uses
- Considered for:
  - patients who can't tolerate ACE inhibitors or angiotensin-II receptor blockers
  - patients already on β-blockers and well controlled:
    - patients with symptomatic angina or a previous heart attack
    - patients exhibiting abnormally high cardiovascular sympathetic tone
    - younger patients, e.g. women intending to have children
    - available as tablets or as injections in some cases.

Adverse effects[‡]
- Fatigue.
- Coldness in extremities, e.g. fingers, toes.
- Dizziness, weakness.
- Dry mouth, skin and eyes.

---

* SLE: Systemic lupus erythematosus, an autoimmune disease.
† There are very many more.
‡ Not comprehensive.

- Less commonly: swelling of hands and/or feet, insomnia, nightmares, wheezing, nausea, vomiting, skin rashes, constipation, depression, impotence.

Precautions and contraindications
- Wean patients off β-blockers gradually.
- Consider not withdrawing β-blockers in patients with a history of myocardial infarction with symptomatic angina unless absolutely necessary.
- β-blockers are absolutely contraindicated in asthmatic patients.
- Avoid use of β-blockers with patients on thiazides due to danger of developing diabetes.
- Other contraindications:
  - uncontrolled heart failure
  - severe bradycardia
  - hypotension
  - Prinzmetal's angina.[*]

α-BLOCKERS
Examples
- Doxazocin.
- Prazocin.
- Indoramin.
- Terazocin.

Mechanism of action
- Block binding of norepinephrine to α-adrenoceptors in peripheral arteriolar walls, causing vasodilatation and lowered TPR.[†]

Uses
- Not the drug of choice due to several adverse effects; may be used together with other antihypertensives in cases of resistant hypertension.
- Available as oral tablets.

Adverse effects
- May precipitate rapid, severe fall in blood pressure with first dose; introduce with great caution.
- Postural hypotension.
- Oedema.
- Dizziness.
- Insomnia.
- Less frequently: hepatitis, diarrhoea, blurred vision, thrombocytopaenia.

---

[*] Prinzmetal's angina: unusual form of angina caused by total occlusion of proximal coronary arteries due to spasm.
[†] TPR: total peripheral resistance.

Precautions and contraindications[*]

- Introduce with caution.
- Avoid use if possible in pregnant or breast-feeding patients.
- Avoid if possible in depressed patients and patients with Parkinson's disease.
- Avoid in patients with heart failure caused by mechanical obstruction, e.g. aortic stenosis (especially prazocin).

DIRECT VASODILATORS

- Dilate blood vessels.
- All act directly on smooth muscle wall to relax it and cause vasodilation.
- Examples: diazoxide, hydralazine, sodium nitroprusside, minoxidil, bosentan, epoprostenol (prostacyclin), iloprost, sildenafil (Viagra), sitaxentan.

Mechanism of action

- Bosentan: binds to and blocks specifically endothelial ET_A and ET_B receptors in smooth muscle, thereby preventing the vasoconstrictor endothelin-1 (ET-1) from binding and constricting the vessel.
- Diazoxide: a K^+-channel activator that increases membrane permeability to K^+ ions, turning off voltage-gated Ca^{2+} ion channels.
- Hydralazine: a powerful vasodilator that inhibits membrane-bound enzymes involved in production of free radicals, which normally block nitric oxide-induced vasodilation.
- Sodium nitroprusside: a source of nitric oxide that dilates blood vessels.
- Minoxidil: a pro-drug, converted *in vivo* to the active sulphated form. Minoxidil sulphate acts by opening membrane-bound adenosine triphosphate-sensitive K^+ channels in arterioles.
- Epoprostenol (Flolan® GSK): a proprietary form of prostacyclin, which is naturally produced in endothelial cells from prostaglandin H_2 to form prostacyclin PGI_2. PGI_2 activates a specific cell-surface receptor (IP receptor, IPR) coupled to adenylate cyclase through G(s)-protein, resulting in vasodilation. Used mainly as an anticoagulant.
- Iloprost: a synthetic analogue of PGI_2. Selectively inhibits cGMP-specific phosphodiesterase type 5, resulting in elevated intracellular concentrations of cyclic AMP, with consequent vasodilation.
- Sitaxentan: a powerful ET-1 receptor antagonist (*see* Bosentan).

---

[*] Not comprehensive; *see* BNF for more details.

Uses

- Diazoxide: hypertensive emergencies; IV injection.
- Hydralazine: hypertensive emergencies; moderate to severe hypertension; oral tablets; IV injection.
- Sodium nitroprusside: hypertensive crisis; use under anaesthesia to maintain controlled hypotension; in acute and chronic heart failure; IV injection or infusion.
- Minoxidil: severe hypertension, together with a diuretic and a β-blocker; oral tablets.
- Bosentan: pulmonary arterial hypertension;* oral tablets.
- Epoprostenol: primary pulmonary hypertension resistant to other treatments; also given to inhibit platelet aggregation during kidney dialysis; powder for reconstitution and IV infusion.
- Iloprost: pulmonary arterial hypertension; inhalation nebuliser.
- Sildenafil: pulmonary arterial hypertension; erectile dysfunction; oral tablets.
- Sitaxentan: pulmonary arterial hypertension; oral tablets.

Adverse effects†

- Diazoxide: most commonly hyperglycaemia, hypotension, tachycardia, H_2O and Na^+ retention; less commonly, hirsutism, leucopaenia (low white cell count), thrombocytopaenia (low platelet count), cardiomegaly (heart enlargement).
- Hydralazine: many reported; cardiovascular and blood disturbances, e.g. arrhythmias, hypotension, leukocytopaenia, thrombocytopaenia; CNS: agitation, anxiety, syncope, dizziness; GIT upsets; neuromuscular disturbances, e.g. myalgia, neuralgia.
- Sodium nitroprusside: dramatic hypotension caused by too-rapid infusion: symptoms include nausea, vomiting, syncope, dizziness, headache, arrhythmias (palpitations); remedy: reduce infusion rate; symptoms also of the toxic metabolite viz. cyanide.
- Minoxidil: hypertrichosis (excessive hair growth), tachycardia, peripheral oedema and weight gain.
- Bosentan: cardiovascular: hypotension, arrhythmias (palpitations), flushing; GIT: dry mouth, liver impairment; immune system: hypersensitivity reactions: anaphylaxis, pruritis, skin rashes.
- Epoprostenol: hypotension, bradycardia, hyperglycaemia, chest pain.
- Iloprost: hypotension, chest pain, nausea.

---

* Pulmonary arterial hypertension: high blood pressure in the pulmonary artery or lung vasculature, causing shortness of breath, dizziness and syncope.
† Not comprehensive; see BNF for more details.

- Sildenafil: insomnia, pyrexia, vasodilatation (used in treatment of erectile dysfunction).
- Sitaxentan: reversible induction of liver microsomal enzymes, GIT upsets, oedema, increased INR.[*]

Precautions and contraindications[†]

- Diazoxide:
    - precautions: to be used with caution if at all during pregnancy and labour
    - contraindications: in patients with ischaemic heart disease and kidney disease; reflex sympathetic response to diazoxide can trigger angina and cardiac failure.
- Hydralazine:
    - precautions include: liver or kidney disease, cerebrovascular or coronary heart diseases, pregnancy, breast-feeding
    - contraindications include: systemic lupus erythematosus (SLE; lupus), cor pulmonale;[‡] porphyria,[§] myocardial insufficiency through mechanical obstruction, aortic aneurism (balloon-like swelling in the aortic wall).
- Sodium nitroprusside:
    - precautions include: increased intracranial pressure; liver disease; pregnancy and breast-feeding – little data available; best to avoid if possible in pregnant or nursing mothers; under anaesthesia patient's ability to control hypovolaemia and anaemia already reduced by the anaesthetic
    - contraindications include: patients with acute congestive heart failure and reduced TPR; surgery in patients known to have an inadequate cerebral circulation; do not use to treat compensatory hypertension in patients with arteriovenous shunting or aortic coarctation.

ACE INHIBITORS
Examples

- Captopril.
- Enalapril.
- Cilazapril.
- Lisinopril.

---

[*] INR: International Normalization Ratio: a measurement of blood clotting time increase with an oral anticoagulant.
[†] Not comprehensive.
[‡] Cor pulmonale: enlargement of the right ventricle of the heart through disease of the lungs or of the pulmonary blood vessels.
[§] Porphyria: hereditary disease caused by failure to synthesise haem, with urinary excretion of porphyrins, causing reddish urine colour (disease of King George III).

Mechanism of action

- Block angiotensin-converting enzyme (ACE) which catalyses conversion of inactive angiotensin-I to active angiotensin-II.

Uses

- Good first treatment choice in young Caucasians; response is poorer in older (> 55 years) patients and in Afro-Caribbean patients.
- Generally a good choice for patients with insulin-dependent diabetes mellitus with nephropathies that cause proteinurea and microalbuminuria.*
- Also used as prophylaxis against stroke in patients after myocardial infarction.
- Available as oral tablets.

Adverse effects

- Severe hypotension.
- Persistent dry cough.
- Delayed onset angioedema,† especially in Afro-Caribbean patients.
- Skin rashes.
- GIT symptoms including nausea, vomiting, constipation and diarrhoea.
- Others reported include dizziness, headache, fatigue, taste disturbances and bronchospasm.

Precautions and contraindications

- Use with care in patients on diuretics due to sudden volume loss and drastic fall in blood pressure.
- Use with care in patients with any renal disease and monitor renal function before and during treatment with ACE inhibitors.
- Use with care in patients with aortic stenosis due to danger of hypotension.
- Monitor patients carefully if mixing ACE inhibitors with any other diuretics (best to avoid this combination if possible).
- Perhaps best avoided during breast-feeding.
- ACE inhibitors are contraindicated during pregnancy and in patients who have shown previous hypersensitivity to them.
- ACE inhibitors are contraindicated in patients with renovascular disease.

---

* Microalbuminuria: very small increase in urinary albumin; indicative of early stage of kidney malfunction.
† Angioedema: swellings below the skin due to oedema, often around the eyes and mouth.

ANGIOTENSIN-II RECEPTOR BLOCKERS (ARBS)
Examples
- Candesartan.
- Irbesartan.
- Olmesartan.
- Eprosartan.
- Losartan.
- Telmisartan.

Mechanism of action
- Block the binding of angiotensin-II to the AT-II receptor, thereby blocking the effects of angiotensin-II.

Uses
- Alternative therapy to ACE inhibitors with hypertensive patients who cannot tolerate ACE inhibitors.
- For patients who need treatment for heart failure or diabetic nephropathy.

Adverse effects
- Generally milder than for ACE inhibitors.
- Angioedema.
- Dizziness (the most frequent adverse effect, through hypotension); more common with patients on diuretics.
- Hyperkalaemia.
- Musculoskeletal pain.
- Nausea and vomiting.

Precautions and contraindications
- Use with caution in patients:
  - with renal problems, especially renal arterial stenosis
  - who are hyperkalaemic
  - with aortic or mitral valve stenosis
  - who are Afro-Caribbean (ARBs may not be effective).
- ARBS are contraindicated in:
  - pregnancy and during breast-feeding
  - biliary obstruction, cirrhosis (valsartan).

CALCIUM CHANNEL BLOCKERS
Examples
- Amlopidine.
- Felodipine.
- Lacidipine.
- Nicardipine.
- Diltiazem.
- Isradipine.
- Lercanidipine.
- Nifedipine.

- Nimodipine.
- Verapamil.

- Nisoldipine.

Mechanism of action

- Ca^{2+}-channel blockers act by blocking L-type voltage-gated Ca^{+2} channels in blood vessels and the heart.

Uses

- Treatment of angina* and arrhythmias, e.g. verapamil.[†]
- Treatment of hypertension, e.g. amlopidine, diltiazem, felodipine, isradipine.
- Prophylaxis against or treatment of spasms resulting from brain haemorrhage, e.g. nimodipine.

Adverse effects[‡]

- Generally those usually associated with vasodilation, e.g. headaches, flushing, syncope; also, to a greater or lesser extent:
  - bradycardia
  - ankle oedema
  - sino-atrial and AV block
  - nausea
  - dizziness (the most frequent adverse effect, through hypotension); more common with patients on diuretics
  - hyperkalaemia
  - musculoskeletal pain
  - nausea and vomiting
  - hepatic or renal problems (rarely)
  - some reports of angina exacerbation after withdrawal of treatment.

Precautions and contraindications[§]

- Avoid grapefruit juice which affects metabolism of some of the Ca^{2+}-channel blockers.
- Kidney or liver impairment.
- Myocardial infarction, especially with verapamil.
- Pregnancy.
- Impaired left ventricular function.
- Patients with cerebral oedema, especially with nimodipine.
- Patients on β-blockers, especially with verapamil.

---

* Especially when angina is associated with coronary vasospasm.
† But avoid verapamil or diltiazem use in patients with heart failure as they depress cardiac function.
‡ Not comprehensive; *see* BNF for more details about each drug.
§ Not comprehensive; examples given for rapid study only; readers who need more information should consult colleagues and authoritative texts before prescribing.

Chapter 26 Quiz

ANSWER T (TRUE) OR F (FALSE)

1. Treat with antihypertensives if BP 140/90 + no organ damage + no cardiovascular complications. ☐
2. Lifestyle counselling advice involves:
   Weight reduction. ☐
   Exercise if possible. ☐
   Reduce salt, alcohol and fatty food intake. ☐
   Stop smoking. ☐
3. The aims of drug treatment are:
   In most cases to keep blood pressure below 140/90 mmHg. ☐
   For diabetics or patients with renal disease, below 120/80. ☐
4. Drugs used include:
   Aspirin. ☐
   Thiazide diuretics. ☐
   Heparin. ☐
   ACE inhibitors. ☐
   Angiotensin-II receptor antagonists. ☐
   Calcium channel blockers. ☐
   Centrally acting drugs, e.g. clonidine. ☐
   Direct vasodilators. ☐
   β-adrenoceptor agonists. ☐
5. For young white patients, ACE inhibitors are initial choices. ☐
6. ACE inhibitors may not be effective in Black patients initially. ☐
7. β-blockers are favoured initially for uncomplicated hypertension. ☐
8. Diltiazem and verapamil are usually suitable for angina patients. ☐
9. α-blockers are used only in very resistant cases of hypertension. ☐
10. ARBs are useless in patients intolerant to ACE inhibitors. ☐
11. Thiazide diuretics inhibit Na^+/Cl^- reabsorption in distal tubules. ☐
12. Thiazides are often first line of treatment in newly diagnosed hypertension. ☐
13. Thiazides may cause hyperglycaemia and hyperuricaemia. ☐
14. Thiazides should not be used in patient's with Addison's disease. ☐
15. β-blockers are contraindicated in:
    Asthmatic patients. ☐
    Uncontrolled heart failure. ☐

Hypotension. ☐

Prinzmetal's angina. ☐

16. Direct vasodilators stimulate ACh receptors on smooth muscle. ☐

17. Adverse effects with hydralazine include:

Arrhythmias. ☐

Hypotension. ☐

Thrombocytopaenia. ☐

Leucopaenia. ☐

Hair loss. ☐

18. Sodium nitroprusside can cause precipitous hypotension. ☐

19. ACE inhibitors are:

A good first line treatment with young Caucasians. ☐

Favoured for patients with IDDM and nephropathies. ☐

Prophylactic against stroke after myocardial infarction. ☐

Available only in injectable form. ☐

Contraindicated in patients with renovascular disease. ☐

20. Angiotensin-II receptor blockers include:

Candesartan. ☐

Eprosartan. ☐

Captopril. ☐

21. Calcium channel blockers include:

Amlopidine. ☐

Diltiazem. ☐

Nifedipine. ☐

Verapamil. ☐

Nicorandil. ☐

22. Ca^{2+}-channel blockers block L-type voltage-gated Ca^{2+} channels. ☐

23. Ca^{2+}-channel blockers are used as prophylaxis against angina. ☐

24. Ca^{2+}-channel blockers are used to treat hypertension, e.g. diltiazem. ☐

25. Ca^{2+}-channel blockers may cause bradycardia and syncope. ☐

27 Inflammation I: introduction

Learning objectives ■ A definition of inflammation ■ Phases of inflammation ■
Some important chemical mediators of inflammation ■ Hypersensitivity reactions
■ Important drug strategies when treating inflammation

Learning objectives
- Know what is meant by the acute and chronic phases of inflammation.
- Be able to list some important mediators of inflammation.
- Be able to give examples of the different types of hypersensitivity.
- Know the current main approaches to drug treatment of inflammatory disorders.

A definition of inflammation
- Protective molecular and cellular responses to harmful stimuli.

Phases of inflammation
- Acute: initial tissue defensive response to:
    - pathogens, e.g. bacteria and viruses
    - neoplastic cells
    - harmful chemicals or ionising radiation
    - physical trauma, e.g. wounding, frostbite
    - aims to keep tissue damage localised and eradicate it.
- Chronic: persistent inflammation involving:
    - tissue destruction
    - angiogenesis
    - fibrosis
    - medical problems such as rheumatoid arthritis.

Some important chemical mediators of inflammation*
- Histamine.
- Opsonins,† e.g. C3a, which stimulates histamine release from mast cells.
- 5-hydroxytryptamine (5-HT; serotonin).
- Prostaglandins.
- Leukotrienes.

---

* Not comprehensive.
† Opsonin: a serum chemical that adheres to invading organisms, for example bacteria and attracts phagocytes.

- Bradykinin.
- Tumour necrosis factor-α (TNF-α).

Inflammatory responses are often in response to hypersensitivity reactions. For a summary of some important inflammatory pathways and sites of anti-inflammatory drug action *see* Figure 27.1.

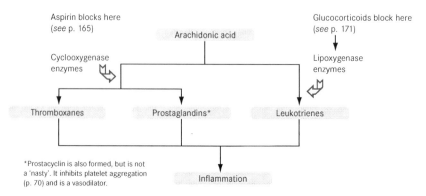

FIGURE 27.1A Sites of action of aspirin and glucocorticoids.

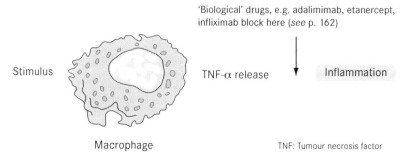

FIGURE 27.1B Sites of action of some 'biological' drugs.

HYPERSENSITIVITY REACTIONS

Type 1 Allergic reactions

- Reactions to eggs, bee stings, with release of mediators: histamine, prostaglandins, leukotrienes, 5-HT.
- Consequences:
    - local, e.g. oedema, itching, rhinitis (hay fever, inflammation of nasal mucous membranes)
    - systemic: anaphylactic shock (generalised histamine release and profound, possibly fatal, fall in blood pressure).
- Treatment includes:

   + topical or systemic antihistamines
   + topical or systemic corticosteroids
   + epinephrine (By IV injection or infusion in anaphylactic shock to raise blood pressure and stimulate the heart) + O_2 if available and artificial ventilation.

Type 2: Antibody-mediated

- Graves' disease (*see* also Type 5); hyperthyroidism when circulating antibodies bind to the TSH receptor and stimulate excessive thyroid release:
  - treatment includes:
    + anti-thyroid drugs
    + partial thyroid ablation.
- Hashimoto's thyroiditis (hypothyroidism when circulating antibodies attack and destroy thyroid cells):
  - treatment (mainly):
    + replacement treatment with thyroxine.

Type 3: Immune complex deposition

- The Arthus reaction (delayed tissue reaction after, e.g. vaccination, with symptoms after 4–12 hours of pain, swelling, oedema, haemorrhage, and necrosis.
- Glomerulonephritis (kidney disease).
- Rheumatoid arthritis.
- Systemic lupus erythematosus (SLE; lupus).

Type 4: Cell-mediated

- Due to contact with, e.g. nickel in watchstraps, poison ivy, hair colourings, rubber gloves; symptoms generally appear after 2–4 days.
- Treatment:
  + identify irritant
  + drugs include: topical or systemic steroids (mainly anti-inflammatory), azathioprine, immunosuppressants, cyclosporine, soothing creams.

Type 5:* Stimulatory

Hypersensitivity reaction caused by antibody reactions with cell surface receptors, for example:
- Graves' disease (*see* Type 2).

---

* Some authorities classify Graves' disease as Type 2; both options are given here.

- Myasthenia gravis (muscle paralysis due to circulating antibodies to the nicotinic ACh receptor on skeletal muscle).
- Symptoms:
  - ◆ muscle weakness and progressive paralysis.
- Treatment includes:
  - ◆ anticholinesterases to potentiate ACh activity at the receptor
  - ◆ immunosuppressants to suppress antibody production
  - ◆ thymectomy in some cases.

Classification note: Type 5 is pretty much a British classification; most other countries stick with Types 1–4.

Important drug strategies when treating inflammation

- Treat pain and inflammation by blocking synthesis of pain-producing mediators with non-steroidal anti-inflammatory drugs, e.g. aspirin, paracetamol, celecoxib.
- Suppress immune responses and block inflammatory reactions with synthetic corticosteroids e.g. prednisolone.
- Slow disease progression with 'biological' drugs, e.g. etanercept, infliximab, which block key mediators of the inflammatory response, e.g. TNF-α.

Chapter 27 Quiz

ANSWER T (TRUE) OR F (FALSE)

1. Inflammation is the tissue response to damaging stimuli. ☐
2. Inflammation has two phases, acute and chronic. ☐
3. The acute phase involves angiogenesis and tissue destruction. ☐
4. Important chemical mediators of inflammation include:
   Histamine. ☐
   5-HT. ☐
   Norepinephrine. ☐
   Prostaglandins. ☐
   Leukotrienes. ☐
   TNF-α. ☐
5. Type I hypersensitivity:
   Is antibody-mediated. ☐

Chemical mediators include histamine and 5-HT. ☐

Reactions present with, for example, oedema, hay fever and itch. ☐

Can result in anaphylactic shock. ☐

Reactions may be treated with antihistamines. ☐

6. Type 2 hypersensitivity:

Is antibody-mediated. ☐

Causes thyroid problems. ☐

7. Type 3 hypersensitivity:

Involves deposition in tissue of immune complexes. ☐

Mediates the Arthus reaction. ☐

Mediates reactions to poison ivy. ☐

Mediates rheumatoid arthritis. ☐

28 Inflammation II: non-steroidal anti-inflammatory drugs (NSAIDs), mainly aspirin

Learning objectives ■ Brief history ■ Classification of NSAIDs with examples ■ Chemistry of aspirin ■ Mechanism of action of aspirin ■ Uses of aspirin and other NSAIDs ■ Aspirin preparations ■ Absorption, metabolism and excretion of aspirin ■ Adverse effects of aspirin and other NSAIDs ■ Precautions and contraindications with NSAIDs

Learning objectives
- Be able to give some examples of NSAIDs.
- Be able to draw the chemical structure of aspirin.
- Know basically how aspirin works.
- Be ready to list uses of NSAIDs.
- Know the forms of aspirin used, the routes of administration of aspirin and the advantages and disadvantages of these routes.
- Be able to give an account of the adverse effects of aspirin and other NSAIDs.
- Know the given precautions and contraindications with NSAIDs.

Brief history
Willow bark has been chewed by people for more than 2000 years, especially by women in labour, and eighteenth century English practitioners, notably Edward Stone, used willow bark to lower fever. Patients were eating salicin, a glycoside, and at the turn of the twentieth century the Bayer Pharmaceutical Company marketed their synthetic derivative, acetylsalicylic acid, under the trade name aspirin.

Classification of NSAIDs with examples
- COX-2 inhibitors:
  - celecoxib
  - etoricoxib
  - lumiracoxib.

- Salicylates:
  - aspirin.
- Arylpropionic acids:
  - fenoprofen
  - ibuprofen
  - ketoprofen.
- Arylalkanoic acids:
  - etodolac
  - indometacin.
- Fenamic acids:
  - mefenamic acid.
- Oxicams:
  - meloxicam
  - piroxicam.

Chemistry of aspirin

Aspirin is acetylsalicylic acid.

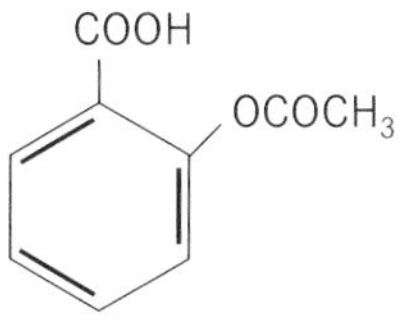

FIGURE 28.1 Aspirin.

Mechanism of action of aspirin

Inhibits cyclooxegenase enzymes (COX-1 and COX-2) in prostaglandin and thromboxane synthesis.

Uses of aspirin and other NSAIDs[*]

Symptomatic relief of inflammation and pain in, for example:
- Bone pain (e.g. metastatic bone pain).
- Fever (pyrexia; raised body temperature).
- Headaches.
- Osteoarthritis.
- Psoriatic arthritis.
- Rheumatoid arthritis.
- Rheumatic fever (aspirin).

---

[*] Note: paracetamol is sometimes mistakenly grouped with NSAIDs. It has little if any anti-inflammatory action.

Also used to treat heart disease:
* Acute myocardial infarction (MI).
* Prophylactic for MI (low doses, e.g. 75 mg).
* Prophylactic for stroke.
* Coronary artery disease.
* Pericarditis.

Aspirin preparations
* Oral: tablets 75 or 300 mg, soluble aspirin, enteric coated aspirin.
* Rectal: suppositories.

Absorption, metabolism and excretion of aspirin[*]
Absorption:
* Stomach: very acidic environment therefore good absorption (aspirin pKA = 3.5); unionised molecules pass more easily across biological membranes; aspirin is a weak acid, therefore poorly ionised in stomach; (*see* Figure 28.2).
* Small intestine: alkaline; good absorption (large surface area despite greater ionisation of aspirin).[†]
* Rectal: good absorption; sidesteps first pass metabolism.

Distribution:
* In plasma, aspirin is hydrolysed to salicylate, which binds to plasma albumin; consequently:
  * plasma half-life increases
  * albumin-salicylate complex may become an antigen and produce hypersensitivity reactions to aspirin.

Metabolism and excretion:
* ± 25% of aspirin is oxidized; some becomes conjugated in liver to glucuronides and excreted in faeces.
* Some salicylate is excreted in urine, especially if urine is alkaline therefore charged; consequently less able to be reabsorbed in the nephron. This is important with aspirin poisoning, since patients should be alkalised to speed up aspirin removal.

Adverse effects of aspirin and other NSAIDs
* GIT effects
  * GIT bleeding
  * dyspepsia ⎤ At therapeutic concentrations
  * gastric ulceration. ⎦

---

[*] Many other NSAIDs share these properties with aspirin.
[†] Reminder: unionised substances cross membranes more easily than do ionised substances.

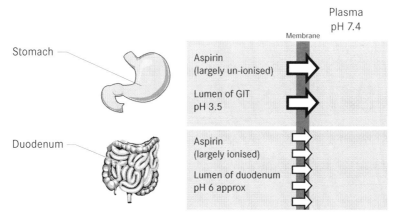

FIGURE 28.2 Effect of pH on absorption of aspirin.

- Renal effects (Not comprehensive; prostaglandins (Pgs) are important in maintenance of normal renal vasodilation and NSAIDs inhibit Pg production):
  - acute renal failure
  - fluid and salt retention
  - tubular necrosis (tissue death)
  - interstitial nephritis (destruction of kidney-supporting tissues).
- Cardiovascular effects include:
  - risk of myocardial infarction, including with COX-2-selective NSAIDs.
- Photosensitivity.

Precautions and contraindications with NSAIDs

- Pregnancy: caution is recommended, especially in the third trimester, when avoidance is usually advisable due to risk of premature closure of a duct, the ductus arteriosis, that keeps blood away from the foetal lungs, which are already fluid-filled (paracetamol is an alternative for pain).
- Gastric and duodenal ulcers: patients with these should consult their practitioner before taking NSAIDs.

Chapter 28 Quiz

ANSWER T (TRUE) OR F (FALSE)

1. Aspirin is anti-inflammatory by stimulating biosynthesis of prostaglandins. ☐
2. NSAIDs are used to treat symptomatic pain and inflammation. ☐
3. Aspirin is poorly absorbed rectally in suppository form. ☐
4. NSAIDs are used to treat arthritic pain. ☐
5. Aspirin is contraindicated for patients at risk of heart diseases. ☐
6. Aspirin is relatively well absorbed from the stomach. ☐
7. Aspirin is well absorbed from the small gut despite the alkaline pH. ☐
8. Aspirin is largely reabsorbed from alkaline urine. ☐
9. At therapeutic doses aspirin causes GIT bleeding. ☐
10. Acute renal failure is an adverse effect of aspirin. ☐
11. There is risk of myocardial infarction with NSAIDs. ☐
12. NSAIDs are best avoided during the third trimester of pregnancy. ☐

29 Inflammation III: steroidal anti-inflammatory drugs

Learning objectives ■ Glucocorticoids ■ Normal control of cortisol synthesis and release from the adrenal cortex ■ Anti-inflammatory actions of synthetic glucocorticoids ■ Mechanism of action of glucocorticoids ■ Examples of inflammatory and autoimmune disorders treated with glucocorticoids ■ Medical use of glucocorticoids

Learning objectives
- Know the names of the three principal natural glucocorticoids given.
- Be able to describe briefly the normal control of cortisol synthesis and release.
- Be able to summarise the anti-inflammatory actions of glucocorticoids.
- Be aware of the adverse effects associated with prolonged use of high dose glucocorticoids.
- Know that withdrawal from prolonged-use glucocorticoid therapy must be gradual and why.

Glucocorticoids
- Natural: involved in regulation of the body's CHO, fat and protein utilisation and response to stress:
  - cortisol –most potent natural glucocorticoid (*see* Figure 29.1)
  - cortisone
  - corticosterone.
- Synthetic: powerful anti-inflammatory properties (for example):
  - beclomethasone (inhaled)
  - betamethasone
  - dexamethasone (*see* Figure 29.1)
  - fludrocortisone
  - hydrocortisone
  - prednisolone
  - prednisone
  - triamcinolone.

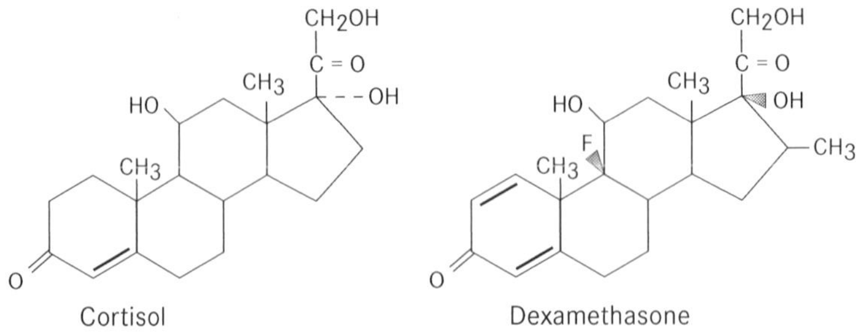

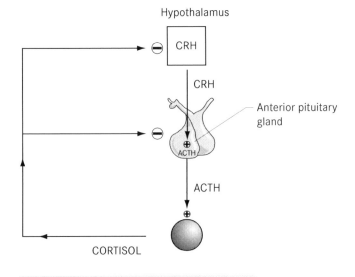

FIGURE 29.1 Structures of cortisol and dexamethasone.

Normal control of cortisol synthesis and release from the adrenal cortex

- Hypothalamic CRH releases anterior pituitary ACTH.
- ACTH stimulates adrenocortical cortisol synthesis and release.
- Cortisol negative feedback to hypothalamus and anterior pituitary to limit further cortisol release.

FIGURE 29.2 Negative feedback control by cortisol.

Anti-inflammatory actions of synthetic glucocorticoids

▪ Inhibition of eiconasoid, e.g. prostaglandin synthesis.
▪ Inhibition of tissue inflammatory processes by activating lipocortin, which:
  ▪ binds to leukocyte membrane receptors, and
  ▪ inhibits inflammatory reactions (for example):
    ♦ chemotaxis
    ♦ phagocytosis
    ♦ release of inflammatory mediators, e.g. cytokines.

Mechanism of action of glucocorticoids

▪ Cortisol being an uncharged molecule diffuses out of the bloodstream and into the cell.
▪ Cortisol binds to a specific intracellular receptor in the cytoplasm or in the nucleus.
▪ The cortisol-receptor complex binds to DNA and alters gene expression.
▪ The newly synthesised mRNA moves to the cytoplasm where it is translated into new proteins.

Examples of inflammatory and autoimmune disorders treated with glucocorticoids

▪ Rheumatoid arthritis.
▪ Systemic lupus erythematosus (lupus; SLE).
▪ Psoriasis.
▪ Asthma.
▪ Eczema.
▪ Non-disease-related joint inflammation through, e.g. sport, injury.

Medical use of glucocorticoids

▪ Administration:
  ▪ oral tablets, e.g. betamethasone, dexamethasone
  ▪ inhalation, e.g. beclomethasone
  ▪ injection into joints, IM
  ▪ topical, e.g. hydrocortisone.
▪ Patients on prolonged high dose glucocorticoids need:
  ▪ to increase the dose at the doctor's discretion if they become ill, and depending on the severity of the illness
  ▪ before an operation to inform, if they are able, the anaesthetist and surgeon that they are on high glucocorticoid therapy. The referring GP should inform the surgical team
  ▪ regular monitoring for adverse effects.

- Adverse effects with prolonged use of high doses; patient develops symptoms similar to those of Cushing's disease:
  - atrophy (wasting) of the adrenal cortex
  - bone thinning and osteoporosis
  - carbohydrate metabolism disturbances
  - diabetes
  - electrolyte imbalances with sodium retention and oedema (swollen ankles and 'moon face')
  - euphoria
  - growth retardation in children
  - gastric ulcers
  - hirsutism
  - hypertension
  - immune reactions suppressed
  - infections may be masked
  - muscle wasting
  - striae (stretch marks on skin)
  - suppression of the adrenocortical axis and of normal stress responses
  - osteoporosis
  - redistribution of body fat, e.g. hump on the back.
- Withdrawal of glucocorticoids:
  - must be gradual due to the complete suppression of the normal CRH-ACTH-corticosteroid axis by prolonged high dose glucocorticoids
  - abrupt withdrawal leaves the patient susceptible to stress, e.g. infection, injury
  - doses of glucocorticoid are tapered with time to allow recovery of the physiological control systems.

Chapter 29 Quiz

ANSWER T (TRUE) OR F (FALSE)

1. Cortisol is the most potent physiological glucocorticoid. ☐
2. Synthetic glucocorticoids vary in potency. ☐
3. Anti-inflammatory actions of glucocorticoids include:
   Inhibition of prostaglandin synthesis. ☐
   Activating lipocortin. ☐
   Inhibiting release of inflammatory cytokines. ☐
   Promoting phagocytosis. ☐

4. Normal control of cortisol release involves:

   Hypothalamic CRH. ☐

   Which promotes pituitary ACTH release. ☐

   Which promotes adrenal cortisol release. ☐

   Inhibition of CRH and ACTH release by cortisol. ☐

   Which promotes further cortisol release. ☐

5. Anti-inflammatory actions of glucocorticoids involve:

   Inhibition of eiconasoid biosynthesis. ☐

   Inactivation of lipocortin activity. ☐

   Inhibition of chemotaxis. ☐

   Inhibition of phagocytosis. ☐

   Inhibition of inflammatory cytokine release. ☐

6. Cortisol mechanism involves *de novo* protein synthesis. ☐

7. Beclomethasone is available in inhalation form. ☐

8. Glucocorticoids can be administered into an inflamed joint. ☐

9. Glucocorticoids are not taken orally. ☐

10. Patients on high dose glucocorticoids have special requirements (for example):

    Gradual withdrawal from the drug. ☐

    Surgical team prior knowledge that they are on glucocorticoids. ☐

    Possibly higher drug doses when ill. ☐

    Regular monitoring for adverse reactions. ☐

11. Adverse reactions include:

    Hypertrophy of the adrenal cortex. ☐

    Oedema and redistribution of body fat. ☐

    Osteoporosis and bone thinning. ☐

    Suppression of the immune system. ☐

    Depression. ☐

    Suppression of the hypothalamic CRH-ACTH axis. ☐

30 Inflammation IV: disease-modifying anti-rheumatic drugs (DMARDs)

Learning objectives ■ What are DMARDs? ■ Examples of DMARDs ■ Anti-malarial and anti-giardial drugs ■ Drugs that interfere with nucleic acid synthesis ■ Use of folic acid ■ Cytokine inhibitors DMARDs ■ Theoretical background ■ Treatment of autoimmune and inflammatory conditions ■ Adverse reactions reported

Learning objectives

- Know what is meant by DMARDs.
- Be able to give examples of DMARDs and, where known, their mechanism of action and how they are administered.
- Be aware of the adverse effects of DMARDs, which suppress the immune system.
- Be able to explain briefly what a cytokine inhibitor is and give examples.
- Know some of the adverse effects and precautions with cytokine inhibitors.

What are DMARDs?

- Drugs used in an attempt to slow the progression of progressively disabling conditions (for example):
    - Crohn's disease
    - rheumatoid arthritis
    - systemic lupus erythematosus (lupus; SLE).
    - psoriasis and psoriatic arthritis
    - Sjögren's syndrome*

Examples of DMARDs

- Gold. ⎤
- Penicillamine. ⎦ Becoming obsolete because of adverse effects and better drugs are available; not dealt with here
- Antimalarial drugs: particularly useful in lupus.
- Immune response-modifying drugs (for example):
    - azathioprine ⎤
    - leflunomide ⎥ Interfere with nucleic acid synthesis
    - methotrexate. ⎦

---

* Sjögren's syndrome: an autoimmune disease, causing inflammation of the lachrymal and salivary glands; can be primary or secondary to other problems, for example RA or lupus, and causes dryness in eyes and mouth and may affect mood.

- Cytokine inhibitors (better known as 'biologic' drugs; in the UK sometimes called biological drugs).*

Anti-malarial and anti-giardial† drugs
- Chloroquine.
- Hydroxychloroquine. ⎤ Anti-malarial
- Mepacrine: used to treat the protozoan parasite *Giardia lamblia*, which colonises the intestine; also indicated for lupus.

Mechanism of action
- For malaria, chloroquine allows toxic levels of haem to accumulate in the malarial mosquito parasite, killing it.
- Chloroquine is also used to control SLE, but its mechanism is unknown, although it may act both in the parasite and in lupus patients by inducing nitric oxide. It needs to be taken for some months before lupus patients begin to get the drug's beneficial effect.

Adverse effects
- With chloroquine and other antimalarials, e.g. mepacrine, include visual disturbances with potentially serious corneal deposits and regular visual acuity tests are essential when using these. Other effects include GIT disturbances, hypersensitivity reactions and, relatively rarely, bone marrow depression.

Drugs that interfere with nucleic acid synthesis
- Azathioprine. ⎤
- Leflunomide. ⎬ Interfere with nucleic acid synthesis
- Methotrexate. ⎦

These drugs, also used to treat cancer, are given in far lower doses as anti-rheumatic drugs, either as DMARDs in their own right, or supplementary to other treatments. Methotrexate is prescribed together with infliximab (*see* p. 177) to reduce the body's immune response to the infliximab.

Use of folic acid
- Patients on methotrexate should also be given regular courses of folic acid to protect against GIT upsets associated with DMARDs such as methotrexate.

---

* Biological drugs are also being designed to treat certain cancers (*see* p. 235).
† *Giardia lamblia* is a parasitic protozoan.

Safety note: patients on these and all other DMARDs which depress immune function must be given regular blood platelet, differential white cell and full blood counts.

Cytokine inhibitors (biologic (USA)/biological (UK)) DMARDs

These drugs are part of a rapidly growing armoury of drugs that treat auto-immune disease such as RA, and neoplastic diseases (cancers; *see* p. 235). They have revolutionised the treatment of many inflammatory and autoimmune disorders, such as Crohn's disease and RA due to a reduction in the incidence and severity of pain and the restoration of mobility for the arthritic patient.

Theoretical background

- These drugs are artificially created proteins directed against mediators of the immune response. These mediators include:
  - tumour necrosis factor-α (TNF-α)
  - interleukin-1 (IL-1).

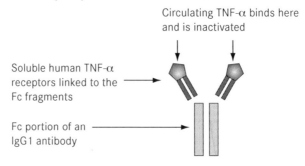

FIGURE 30.1 Structure of etanercept, a cytokine inhibitor ('biological drug').

Treatment of autoimmune and inflammatory conditions

- Adalimumab: blocks TNF-α.
- Anakinra: blocks IL-1.
- Etanercept: blocks TNF-α.
- Infliximab: blocks TNF-α.

Adverse reactions reported (not comprehensive, and not all patients experience these)

- Adalimumab:
  - upper respiratory tract infections
  - reactions at the injection site
  - reports of opportunistic bacterial and fungal infections
  - optic neuritis (inflammation of the optic nerve) exacerbation of myocardial infarction.

* Anakinra:
  * injection site reactions
  * headaches
  * joint or skin infections
  * low white cell counts
  * upper respiratory tract infections.
* Etanercept:
  * injection site reactions
  * upper respiratory tract infections
  * reports of opportunistic bacterial and fungal infections
  * optic neuritis (inflammation of the optic nerve)
  * exacerbation of myocardial infarction.
* Infliximab:
  * anaphylactic reactions with lowered blood pressure, breathing difficulties
  * infusion site reactions
  * lowered white cell count
  * upper respiratory tract infections
  * optic neuritis
  * opportunistic bacterial and fungal reactions.

Safety note: patients should be given tests for TB before starting a course with a cytokine inhibitor. Patients with active TB should not be started on cytokine inhibitors, which lower resistance to infection.

TABLE 30.1 DRUG USE

DETAILS OF USE	ADALIMUMAB	ANAKINRA	ETANERCEPT	INFLIXIMAB
Administration	SC	SC	SC	IV infusion*
Dose frequency	Once every two weeks	Once daily	Once or twice a week	Once every 8 weeks for RA
Half-life of drug	12–14 days	6 hours	5 days	8–10 days
Need for methotrexate	At prescriber's discretion	Not needed	Not needed	Methotrexate needed
Benefit felt after about:	2–4 weeks	4–6 weeks	2–4 weeks	2–4 weeks

* Must be given in a clinical environment by qualified staff with adequate resuscitation facilities

Chapter 30 Quiz

ANSWER T (TRUE) F (FALSE)

1. DMARDs are disease-modifying antirheumatic drugs. ☐
2. Antimalarial drugs are used to treat SLE. ☐
3. Important diseases targeted by DMARDs include:
   Rheumatoid arthritis. ☐
   Crohn's disease. ☐
   Sjögren's syndrome. ☐
   Influenza. ☐
4. DMARDs currently comprise:
   Antimalarial drugs. ☐
   Drugs that interfere with nucleic acid synthesis. ☐
   Drugs that inhibit or block inflammatory cytokines. ☐
   Drugs that primarily block second messengers ☐
5. Gold and penicillamine have been used as DMARDs. ☐
6. Currently used inhibitors of nucleic acid synthesis include:
   Azathioprine. ☐
   Leflunomide. ☐
   Methotrexate. ☐
   Aspirin. ☐
7. Currently used antimalarial drugs include:
   Quinidine. ☐
   Chloroquine. ☐
   Hydroxychloroquine. ☐
   Mepacrine. ☐
8. Patients on antimalarials need regular checks for visual acuity. ☐
9. Nucleic acid inhibitors can depress bone marrow function. ☐
10. Patients on methotrexate should avoid folic acid. ☐
11. Cytokine inhibitors are genetically engineered proteins. ☐
12. Anakinra is designed to inactivate TNF-α. ☐
13. Infliximab is administered by continuous IV infusion. ☐
14. Adalimumab is designed to block TNF-α. ☐
15. Patients on cytokine inhibitors may develop opportunistic fungal or bacterial infections. ☐

31 Inflammation V: gout, scleroderma and Raynaud's phenomenon

Learning objectives ■ Gout ■ Scleroderma ■ Raynaud's phenomenon

Learning objectives

- Be able to give an account of the features of gout.
- Know the names of drugs used to treat gout.
- Be able to list the adverse effects of probenecid.
- Know the given mechanisms of action of probenecid and allopurinol.
- Be able to give a brief classification of the different forms of scleroderma.
- Know what is meant by Raynaud's phenomenon, what may cause it and how it is treated.
- Be able to give a brief account of the treatments for scleroderma.

Gout

- Is an inflammatory reaction to the deposition of uric acid crystals in joint and tendon articular cartilage and tendons.
- Is caused by abnormally slow excretion of urate ion by the kidney; patients may not have abnormally raised urate.
- Occurs more in men than in women, after the age of 40, who may be predisposed to hypertension, type 2 diabetes and cardiac disease.
- Is classically associated with over-indulgence in food and alcohol; obesity may increase the chances of suffering from gout.
- Often occurs in the big toe, where it is called *podagra*; affects other joints, e.g. shoulder, elbow, heel, fingers and wrists.
- Is characterised by symptoms, principally:
  - excruciating, burning pain at sites of urate deposition (*see* Figure 31.1)
  - discharging skin eruptions
  - tophi – swelling caused by gradual build-up of uric acid crystals
  - raised CRP (C-reactive protein), ESR (erythrocyte sedimentation rate) and raised blood viscosity.
- May be secondary to, e.g. kidney disease, and possibly to treatment with diuretics, especially thiazides.

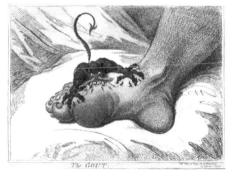

FIGURE 31.1 *Gout* by James Gillray (1799).

Treatment of gout

- NSAIDs for pain alleviation:
  - diclofenac
  - indometacin
  - naproxen
  - ketoprofen.

  Together with a proton pump inhibitor, e.g. omeprazole to protect lining from these drugs
- Colchicine from meadow saffron (*Colchicum autumnale*):
  - in patients who do not respond to NSAIDs
  - acts in gout possibly by blocking migration of neutrophils into the affected joint
  - mechanism is by binding to the intracellular protein tubulin and blocking formation of microtubules
  - adverse effects include diarrhoea, nausea and vomiting
  - contraindicated in pregnancy and used with caution in the elderly and in patients with heart, kidney or GIT disease.
- Uricosuric* drugs for long term management of gout:
  - probenecid
  - sulphinpyrazole

  Promote uric acid excretion in the kidney tubules
  - some adverse effects of probenecid:
    - alopecia (hair loss)
    - anaemia
    - skin rashes
    - GIT upsets
    - nephrotic syndrome (proteinurea, high cholesterol and tissue swelling)
    - pruritis (itching areas)
    - urticaria (itchy wheals).

---

* Uricosuric: promoting uric acid excretion by the kidney.

- Allopurinol:
  - inhibits uric acid synthesis
  - used in patients when probenecid is contraindicated
  - sometimes combined with sulphinpyrazole in resistant cases of gout.

Scleroderma*

- Autoimmune disease caused by hardening of tissues through abnormal overproduction of collagen; the cause is unknown.
- Localised cutaneous (called 'morphoea'):
  - confined mainly to skin of face and neck
  - skin becomes hard and scarred, is scaly and red
  - many patients also develop Raynaud's phenomenon (*see* below).
- Diffuse cutaneous:
  - more widespread, involving the trunk and has a higher incidence of systemic involvement of internal organs.
- Diffuse systemic:
  - affects internal organs, including blood vessels; may not involve skin; sometimes referred to as '*scleroderma sine scleroderma*' (scleroderma without scleroderma)
  - in earlier stages, within the first 10 years, symptoms may be confined to Raynaud's phenomenon; little cutaneous fibrosis and some oesophageal involvement
  - after about 10 years, patients generally develop more serious skin thickening and systemic problems including oesophageal stricture, small bowel malabsorption and pulmonary hypertension. During the last stages there may be widespread deposition of calcium as hydroxyapatite in tissues (calcinosis) with ulcers and severe pulmonary hypertension.

Raynaud's phenomenon

- Is icy coldness in fingers with visible blanching.
- Is caused by spasm of blood vessels supplying the fingers, due to atherosclerosis of the small blood vessels in the fingers.
- Often accompanies scleroderma and other autoimmune disorders, e.g. RA, SLE.
- Can also result from:
  - prolonged use of vibrating tools, e.g. road hammers and drills
  - chemicals, e.g. vinyl chloride contact
  - outdoor work in extremes of cold
  - drugs, e.g. ergot, β-blockers, oral contraceptives.

---

* Highly condensed summary of a serious, complex medical problem.

Treatment of scleroderma

* Localised cutaneous; treatment of Raynaud's phenomenon:
  * vasodilators, e.g. calcium channel antagonists, e.g. felodipine or nifedipine (*see* p. 155)
  * carbonic anhydrase inhibitors, e.g. captopril (*see* p. 153)
  * application of warmth to hands.
* For cutaneous scleroderma:
  * application of moisturising ointments and creams to affected skin
  * dietary supplements of vitamin D and UV light
  * treatment of any oesophageal symptoms
  * infected skin lesions may need antibiotics.
* For diffuse scleroderma:
  * immunosuppressants, e.g. antithymocyte globulin, cyclophosphamide, methotrexate
  * drugs such as omeprazole, a proton pump inhibitor for oesophageal reflux, vasodilators and antiarrhythmic drugs.

Lifestyle changes and support: Lifestyle changes include stopping smoking, changing working conditions if they could exacerbate any Raynaud's symptoms, and use of gloves to keep fingers warm. Patients and families will often need backup from social services, especially in later stages of scleroderma.

Chapter 31 Quiz

ANSWER T (TRUE) OR F (FALSE)

1. Gout is caused by an abnormally slow rate of urate excretion. ☐
2. Gout is an inflammatory reaction to urate deposition. ☐
3. Gout often occurs in the knuckles when it is called *podagra*. ☐
4. Gout is characterised by symptoms including:
   Burning pain at sites of urate deposition. ☐
   Discharging skin eruptions. ☐
   Lowered blood viscosity. ☐
   Raised ESR and CRP. ☐
   Tophi. ☐
5. Treatments for gout include:
   Antibiotics. ☐
   Anti-inflammatory drugs. ☐

Colchicine. ☐

Allopurinol. ☐

Probenecid. ☐

6. Adverse effects of probenecid include:

Hair loss. ☐

Anaemia. ☐

GIT upsets. ☐

Nephrotic syndrome. ☐

Urticaria. ☐

Pruritis. ☐

7. Scleroderma is caused by a bacterial infection. ☐

8. Scleroderma may be:

Localised cutaneous. ☐

Diffuse cutaneous. ☐

Diffuse systemic. ☐

9. Raynaud's phenomenon is extreme cold in fingers. ☐

10. Raynaud's phenomenon may be caused by:

Vasodilation of finger arterioles. ☐

Vinyl chloride. ☐

Occupational damage to hands. ☐

Underlying presence of scleroderma. ☐

11. Treatment of Raynaud's phenomenon includes:

Vasoconstrictors. ☐

Warm gloves. ☐

Changing from jobs that aggravate the problem. ☐

12. Treatment of cutaneous scleroderma includes:

Creams and ointments to soften and moisturise skin. ☐

Dietary supplements of vitamin D. ☐

Treatment of any oesophageal symptoms. ☐

13. Treatment of diffuse advanced scleroderma includes:

Immunosuppressants, e.g. cyclophosphamide. ☐

Anti-thymocyte globulin. ☐

Proton pump inhibitors, e.g. ranitidine. ☐

14. Patients with advanced scleroderma may need antiarrhythmic drugs. ☐

32 Paracetamol (USA: acetaminophen)

Learning objectives ■ Chemistry of paracetamol ■ Theories of mechanism of action of paracetamol ■ Clinical use ■ Paracetamol toxicity

Learning objectives
- Know that paracetamol is structurally similar to aspirin.
- Know its indications for use.
- Be able to list the different preparations of paracetamol.
- Know the maximum safe dose and dose frequency.
- Be aware of the precautions and contraindications for paracetamol.
- Be able to give an account of the consequences of and treatment for paracetamol overdose.

Chemistry of paracetamol
- Chemical name: N-(4-hydroxyphenyl)-ethanamide.
- Synthetic.
- Chemical structure: similar to aspirin (*see* Figure 32.1).

Theories of mechanism of action of paracetamol
- Still unknown at time of writing.
- May inhibit cyclooxegenase (COX-1 and 2) enzymes in tissues where peroxides are low, e.g. in brain and endothelial tissue.
- May inhibit a relatively newly discovered COX-3 enzyme, found only in brain and spinal cord.
- May potentiate the analgesic actions of endogenous cannabinoids.

Clinical use
- Indications:
  - analgesic
  - antipyretic.

Clinical note: paracetamol is not anti-inflammatory.

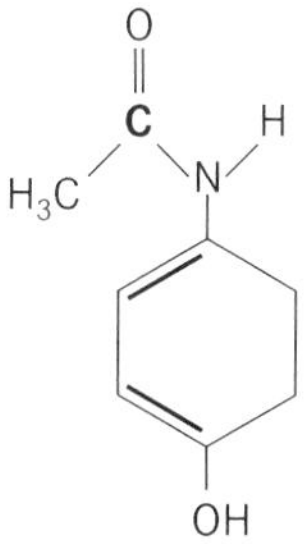

FIGURE 32.1 Paracetamol.

- Preparations:*
  - paracetamol alone:
    - oral tablets 500 mg; paediatric soluble tablets 120 mg
    - suppositories 60 mg, 125 mg and 250 mg
    - oral paediatric solution 120 mg/5 ml
    - IV infusion
  - paracetamol + methionine† (co-methiamol)
  - paracetamol + codeine (co-codamol): paracetamol 100 mg + codeine phosphate 8 mg
  - paracetamol + dextropropoxyfene (co-proxamol): paracetamol 325 mg + dextropropoxyfene HCl 32.5 mg.
- Absorption, metabolism and excretion:
  - well absorbed orally
  - blood levels peak at about 1 hour after administration
  - metabolism by the liver, where paracetamol is:
    - metabolised to a potentially dangerous metabolite, hepatotoxic N-methyl-p-benzoquinone imine, which is
    - rendered harmless by addition of glutathione, and
    - conjugated to produce soluble sulphates and glucuronides
  - excretion is mainly via the kidneys.
- Clinical applications:‡
  - used for:
    - pain
    - mild pyrexia (raised body temperature)
    - brief febrile§ convulsions (diazepam needed for more persistent convulsions)
    - post-immunisation pyrexia (persistent post-immunisation pyrexia requires fast medial assistance)

---

* Not comprehensive; examples given. *See* BNF for more details of preparations.
† Methionine is used as an antidote against paracetamol poisoning.
‡ Not comprehensive.
§ Febrile: feverish.

- ◆ migraine: paracetamol + codeine phosphate + an anti-emetic, e.g. Migraleve® Pfizer
- ◆ use in pregnancy: at time of writing, paracetamol is generally considered the safest analgesic in pregnancy, although use in late pregnancy may be linked to subsequent childhood wheezing.
- ▌ safe doses of paracetamol:
  - ◆ adults: 2 × 500 mg tablets every four hours if required but not to exceed four (4) doses in 24 hours
  - ◆ babies and children: dosage should follow instructions supplied by the manufacturer.
- ▌ adverse effects of paracetamol (rare) include:
  - ◆ skin rashes
  - ◆ leukocytopaenia, thrombocytopaenia
  - ◆ hypotension during an infusion.
- ▌ precautions and contraindications:
  - ◆ alcohol dependence (patient may have damaged liver)
  - ◆ pre-existing liver or kidney damage (paracetamol metabolites are excreted principally via the kidneys).

Paracetamol toxicity

- ▪ Possibly the commonest drug used to induce self-harm in the UK.
- ▪ Limits on number allowed in retail packs (32 tablets per pack in pharmacies).
- ▪ Toxic blood levels:
  - ▌ about 130–150 mg/kg in adults
  - ▌ about 65–75 mg/kg in alcoholics or in cases of malnutrition.
- ▪ Drugs and herbs which increase paracetamol toxicity by inducing hepatic cytochrome P450 metabolising enzymes include:
  - ▌ carbamazepine, phenobarbital, phenytoin (for epilepsy)
  - ▌ rifampicin (an antibiotic)
  - ▌ isoniazid (anti-tubercular drug)
  - ▌ alcohol
  - ▌ hypericum (St John's wort).
- ▪ Other conditions which predispose to paracetamol toxicity include:
  - ▌ genetic factors
  - ▌ malnutrition
  - ▌ being HIV positive.
- ▪ Children are more resistant to paracetamol toxicity.
- ▪ Consequences of paracetamol toxicity:
  - ▌ exhaustion of hepatic glutathione and conjugation system and alternative metabolism of paracetamol to hepatotoxic N–acetyl–*p*–benzoquinone imine (*see* Figure 32.2).

- Symptoms of paracetamol toxicity:
  - asymptomatic for about 24 hours after overdose; there may be nausea and vomiting
  - after about 24 hours symptoms of liver damage can be picked up, e.g.
    - jaundice
    - elevated plasma transaminases, which are liver enzymes released into blood due to liver cell breakdown
    - pain in right upper quadrant (RUQ) of abdomen
    - lactic acidosis (buildup of lactic acid due to the damaged liver's failure to metabolise it)
    - hypoglycaemia (low blood sugar)
    - oliguria (failure of urination); a sign of dehydration
    - kidney failure after 2–3 days.

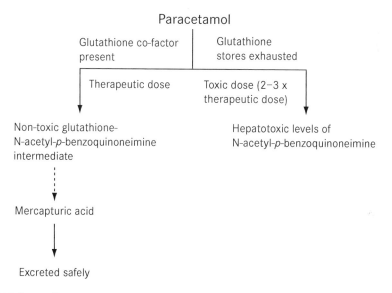

FIGURE 32.2 Paracetamol poisoning.

Treatment of paracetamol poisoning

- Treatment must be initiated as soon as possible.
- Paracetamol levels in blood measured and risk assessed with the help of an appropriate nomogram.[*]
- Oral activated charcoal to adsorb paracetamol before absorption from GIT.
- Acetylcysteine administration by continuous infusion as antidote to toxic

---

[*] Paracetamol nomograms are graphs plotting plasma paracetamol vs. time after ingestion.

metabolite of paracetamol; works by supplying SH groups (normally supplied by glutathione) which inactivate the toxic metabolite.
- Lavage considered if poisoning is life-threatening and is within 60 minutes of taking the overdose; gastric lavage carries a risk of aspiration (secretion of foreign matter into the trachea and lungs).
- If suicide was found to be attempted, the social services may be brought into the case.

Prognosis
Poor if there is:
- renal failure
- severe hepatic encephalopathy
- marked impairment of cognitive function ⎤
- blood pH less than 7.3   ⎬ Liver transplant required
- markedly raised prothrombin time.   ⎦

Chapter 32 Quiz

ANSWER T (TRUE) OR F (FALSE)

1. Paracetamol is prescribed for pain and fever. ☐
2. Paracetamol is similar in structure to aspirin. ☐
3. Paracetamol preparations include:
   Oral tablets 500 mg. ☐
   Suppositories. ☐
   Oral paediatric solution. ☐
   Topical cream. ☐
   Solutions for IV infusion. ☐
4. Paracetamol is highly effective as an anti-inflammatory. ☐
5. Paracetamol may be prescribed for:
   Headache. ☐
   Rheumatic flare-ups. ☐
   Mild pyrexia. ☐
   Migraine. ☐
   Post-immunisation pyrexia. ☐
   Brief febrile convulsions. ☐
6. Adverse effects of paracetamol include skin rashes. ☐
7. Paracetamol is well absorbed orally. ☐

8. Paracetamol is excreted unmetabolised. ☐
9. Is initially metabolised to a toxic intermediate. ☐
10. Which is rendered harmless by addition of liver glutathione. ☐
11. Paracetamol is toxic in overdose due to exhaustion of glutathione. ☐
12. Liver enzyme-inducing drugs enhance paracetamol toxicity. ☐
13. Children are less resistant to paracetamol toxicity. ☐
14. Poisoning is often asymptomatic for the first 24 hours. ☐
15. Symptoms of paracetamol poisoning may include:

    Nausea and vomiting within 24 hours. ☐

    Symptoms of liver damage after 24 hours. ☐

    These symptoms include:

    – jaundice. ☐

    – liver cell enzymes present in the circulation. ☐

    – abdominal pain. ☐

    – hyperglycaemia. ☐

    – oliguria and kidney failure. ☐

16. Treatment includes:

    Oral activated charcoal. ☐

    Acetylcysteine. ☐

33 Opioid analgesics

Learning objectives
- Be able to give an account of the gate theory of pain.
- Be able to use the theory to hypothesise the sites of action of pain-relieving opioids.
- Have a definition for the term 'opioid'.
- Be ready to give examples of endogenous and synthetic opioids.
- Know what is meant by antagonists and partial agonists with examples.
- Be able to list important actions and clinical uses of morphine.
- Know what is meant by tolerance and dependence with regard to opioid abuse and how addicts are helped to get off the drugs.
- Be aware of the properties and uses of methadone.

Perception of pain
- Is perceived by the brain.
- Pain is not felt if nervous pathways carrying pain to the brain are damaged (*see* Figure 33.1).
- The 'gate theory' of pain proposes:*
    - that high intensity stimuli from the body (damaging stimuli) open a 'gate' in the posterior horn of the spinal cord and ascend to the thalamus where the pain is 'felt', and from there to the cerebral cortex where discrimination and interpretation occur
    - that the 'gate' is also controlled by descending impulses from the brain, which decides whether the gate should open or close, which explains how we can be distracted from pain
    - that low intensity ascending impulses unrelated to pain can close the gate and by doing so block pain impulses, which explains how heat therapy at a painful area of the body may ease pain.

---

* The original report: Melzack R, Wall PD. Pain mechanisms: a new theory. *Science*. 1965; **150:** 971–9.

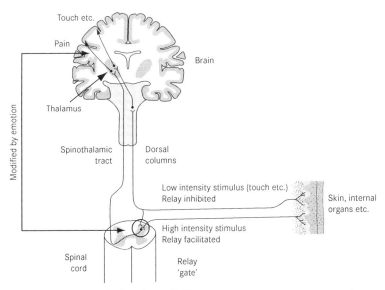

Touch etc.

Pain

Brain

Thalamus

Modified by emotion

Spinothalamic tract

Dorsal columns

Low intensity stimulus (touch etc.)
Relay inhibited

Skin, internal organs etc.

High intensity stimulus
Relay facilitated

Spinal cord

Relay 'gate'

Reproduced with permission from Greenstein BD.
Clinical pharmacology for nurses 17th ed. Churchill Livingstone; 2004

FIGURE 33.1 Pathways involved in perception of pain.

Drugs and the gate theory

▪ Centrally acting pain-relieving drugs, e.g. morphine and other opioids, block pain transmission in the dorsal horn of the spinal cord and the appreciation of pain in higher brain centres.

▪ This suggests that the endogenous opioids are part of the pain gating system.

▪ Local anaesthetics (*see* p. 196) block transmission of pain impulses at the site of tissue damage before they reach the dorsal horn.

Endogenous opioids and opioid pain-relieving drugs

Terminology notes: opioid here is taken to mean any natural or synthetic substance that mimics the actions of morphine and its analogues; a partial agonist is a drug that can act as either an agonist or an antagonist depending on dose.

▪ Endogenous opioids:
  ▪ dynorphins, e.g. dynorphin A
  ▪ encephalins, e.g. metencephalin
  ▪ endorphins, e.g. beta-endorphin.
▪ Examples of agonists:
  ▪ morphine
  ▪ codeine
  } Natural, from opium

- diamorphine (heroin) ⎤
- dihydrocodeine ⎬ Synthetic
- methadone. ⎦
- Examples of partial agonists:
  - buprenorphine
  - meptazinol
  - nalbuphine.
- Antagonists:
  - naloxone
  - naltrexone.

Opioid receptors

- μ_1, μ_2, μ_3 : bind morphine, codeine, encephalins and beta-endorphin; mediate analgesia.
- κ_1, κ_2, κ_3 : bind dynorphins; mediate hallucination.
- δ_1, δ_2: bind encephalins; mediate analgesia and perhaps seizure activity.

Actions of morphine

- Depressant CNS actions:
  - CNS depression
  - depression of pain awareness
  - euphoria
  - analgesia by mimicking endogenous opioid action
  - depression of respiration
  - depression of the cough centre
  - mild hypnotic.
- Stimulant CNS actions:
  - stimulation of nucleus of 3rd nerve results in eye pupil constriction
  - stimulation of chemoreceptor trigger zone results in vomiting
  - stimulation of the vagus nerve, causing slowing of the pulse and lowering blood pressure.

Clinical uses of morphine and other opioids

- Control of pain in (for example):
  - severe pain with anxiety
  - post-operative pain
  - surgical emergencies
  - after an injury
  - control of terminal pain
  - following a coronary thrombosis.
- Diamorphine (heroin):
  - is diacetylmorphine

- crosses the blood–brain barrier faster than morphine and is then converted to morphine
- is more soluble than morphine, produces euphoria faster and is therefore easier to abuse.
- Codeine:
  - has about one-tenth the potency of morphine as a pain suppressant
  - can be taken orally
  - long-established use in cough mixtures; has about one half the potency of morphine in cough suppression
  - constipates.

Adverse effects of morphine and diamorphine

- Depression of respiration, even at therapeutic doses.
- Tolerance and dependence to the central actions of the opioids.
- Sedation.
- Bradycardia (heart slowing).
- Nausea and vomiting.
- Hypersensitivity reactions.
- Confusional states.
- Nightmares.
- Dry mouth.
- Constipation.
- Urinary retention.

Methadone

- Is a synthetic analogue of morphine.
- Has analgesic potency similar to morphine.
- Is well absorbed orally; is not euphoric when taken this way.
- Is euphoric when injected.
- Is used to wean physically dependent patients off heroin.
- Used to be a popular ingredient in cough remedies but withdrawn due to abuse.

Morphine antagonists

- Naloxone and naltrexone.
- Displace morphine and heroin rapidly from their receptors.
- Naloxone works fast when injected SC or IV because it rapidly displaces morphine from its receptor sites. Is used to treat poisoning and overdosing with heroin and morphine.
- Naltrexone is orally absorbed and is used to wean addicts off heroin.

Tolerance and dependence

■ Tolerance is when more of the drug is needed to obtain the same response.

■ Tolerance develops only to the central actions of opioids; therefore doses eventually have to be well beyond normally fatal doses for addicts to obtain the desired effect.

■ Tolerance does NOT develop to peripheral effect of opioids; therefore addicts are chronically severely constipated.

■ Dependence is initially psychological, when the user exhibits drug-seeking behaviour to repeat the euphoria, but can stop without experiencing withdrawal effects.

■ Physical dependence occurs when continual morphine use results in the apparent resetting of the body's autonomic nervous system. This results in extremely unpleasant autonomic responses to the sudden withdrawal of the drug. The user now seeks drugs driven by fear of withdrawal symptoms.

■ Physically dependent addicts need to be weaned gradually off heroin using methadone, for example.

Morphine (and heroin) withdrawal symptoms

■ Restlessness.

■ Yawning.

■ Lacrimation (eyes water).

■ Rhinorrhoea (runny nose).

■ Sweating.

■ Goose flesh ('cold turkey').

■ Abdominal cramps and diarrhoea.

■ Involuntary spasms and leg kicking ('kicking the habit').

■ Vomiting.

■ Heart races (tachycardia).

■ Hyperventilation.

■ Symptoms peak between about 36–72 hours after last 'fix'.

■ 5–7 days to disappearance of symptoms.

■ Craving for drug persists for many months.

■ Relapse is common.

Note: Naloxone administration precipitates withdrawal symptoms immediately.

Chapter 33 Quiz

ANSWER T (TRUE) OR F (FALSE)

1. Pain is perceived at the site of tissue injury. ☐
2. Interruption of nervous afferent pathways can abolish pain perception. ☐
3. Morphine blocks pain at the site of injury. ☐
4. Actions of morphine include:
    CNS depression. ☐
    Depression of pain awareness. ☐
    Depression of respiration. ☐
    Suppression of the cough reflex. ☐
    Hypnotic. ☐
    Euphoria. ☐
    Depression of the vomiting centre. ☐
5. Heroin is diethyl morphine. ☐
6. A partial agonist may, under some conditions, become an antagonist. ☐
7. Codeine is used in cough mixtures. ☐
8. Codeine causes diarrhoea. ☐
9. Heroin does not cross the blood–brain barrier. ☐
10. Tolerance is when more drug is needed to obtain the same response. ☐
11. Psychological dependence is exhibited as drug-seeking behaviour. ☐
12. Physical dependence manifests itself through withdrawal symptoms. ☐
13. Naltrexone is used to wean addicts off morphine or heroin. ☐

34 Local anaesthetics

Learning objectives
- Know the advantages for the patient of local anaesthesia.
- Be able to give examples of local anaesthetics and their uses.
- Know the adverse effects of local anaesthetics.
- Be able to say briefly how they work at the membrane level.

Definition of local anaesthesia
- Loss of all sensation within a circumscribed area of skin or other tissue (e.g. a mucous membrane).

Terminology note: local analgesia is loss of *pain* sensation only.

Local anaesthetics
- Are drugs that produce local anaesthesia.
- Are applied either by topical application or by local injection.
- Have the advantages that:
  - the patient remains conscious and can co-operate if needed
  - they reduce the risks of morbidity and mortality that accompany general anaesthesia
  - they sometimes make hospitalisation unnecessary
  - there are financial advantages for the NHS, but the needs of the patient must come first, for example those who prefer not to be conscious during procedures.

Examples of local anaesthetics
- Cocaine – the prototype, introduced in the UK in 1886; now obsolete and a drug of abuse.
- Bibivucaine.
- Levobibivucaine.
- Lidocaine (lignocaine).
- Novocaine.

- Procaine.
- Ropivacaine.

Use of local anaesthetics (LA)

- Lidocaine is the most commonly used LA.
- It is often formulated with epinephrine for injection because epinephrine constricts local blood vessels and minimises escape of lidocaine into the general circulation and keeps it at the site of injection for longer.
- Local anaesthetics, e.g. lidocaine, may be formulated as gels (used in dentistry; rubbed on gums).
- Lidocaine is used as a gel together with chlorhexidine for urethral catheterisation.
- Lidocaine as an ointment is used to alleviate pain and discomfort for:
  - herpes simplex (e.g. cold sores; genital herpes)
  - herpes zoster (shingles)
  - perineal itching, e.g. pruritus ani
  - epidural injection to reduce the pain of childbirth; a local anaesthetic, often together with an opioid, is injected into the epidural space and blocks passage of nerve impulses.

Adverse effects of local anaesthetics

- Usually due to the escape of the LA into the systemic circulation.
- Cardiovascular complications include: hypotension, bradycardia (slowing of the heart), arrhythmias, ventricular fibrillation, asystole (absence of heartbeat).
- CNS complications include: syncope (fainting), tinnitus (ringing or hissing sounds in the ears), lip and tongue numbness, seizures cardiopulmonary arrest (potentially fatal).
- Hypersensitivity complications (relatively rare) include: oedema, urticaria (itchy rash) at site of injection, anaphylaxis.

Mechanism of action of local anaesthetics

- Blockade of Na^+ channels and thus blockade of impulse conduction along the nerve:
  - the LA exists in the unionised and ionised form on the outer surface of the nerve fibre and the unionised form readily penetrates the fibre to the inner surface of the cell membrane where it is pronated to form an ion
  - the ionised LA binds to the Na^+ channel and blocks it.
- If there is damage and inflammation on the outer surface then the LA will be mainly ionised and therefore less potent.
- The LA binds only to open Na^+ channels and is therefore more potent on rapidly firing neurones.

Chapter 34 Quiz

ANSWER T (TRUE) OR F (FALSE)

1. Local anaesthetics produce a local anaesthesia. ☐
2. Local anaesthesia means a local loss of pain sensation only. ☐
3. Local anaesthetics have the advantage that:
   Patients remain conscious and usually mobile after the procedure. ☐
   Hospitalisation is not always necessary. ☐
   The patient can co-operate during the procedure. ☐
   Fear of general anaesthesia is removed. ☐
4. Examples of local anaesthetics include:
   Bibivucaine. ☐
   Levobibivucaine. ☐
   Lidocaine. ☐
   Procaine. ☐
   Ropivacaine. ☐
5. Lidocaine is often formulated with ACh to constrict local vessels. ☐
6. Local anaesthetics can be applied as gels. ☐
7. Uses for topical application of local anaesthetics include:
   Perineal itching. ☐
   Herpes infections. ☐
   Epidural injections. ☐
8. Adverse effects of local anaesthetics include:
   Hypertension. ☐
   Bradycardia. ☐
   Arrhythmias. ☐
   Dangerous ventricular fibrillation. ☐
   Asystole. ☐
   Tinnitus. ☐
   Seizures. ☐
9. Local anaesthetics block Ca^{2+} channels on the axon membrane. ☐

35 General anaesthetics

Learning objectives ■ A definition of general anaesthesia ■ Before surgery ■ Aims of general anaesthesia ■ The ideal general anaesthetic ■ Stages of general anaesthesia ■ Types of general anaesthetics ■ General anaesthetics administered by inhalation ■ The blood:gas partition coefficient ■ The oil:gas partition coefficient ■ The minimum alveolar concentration (MAC) ■ General anaesthetics administered by injection ■ Muscle relaxants ■ Surgical use ■ Depolarising neuromuscular blocking drugs

Learning objectives

- Know what general anaesthesia is.
- Know the main aims of premedication.
- Be able to list the properties of an ideal general anaesthetic.
- Know the four stages of general anaesthesia.
- Be aware of the main classes of general anaesthetic, i.e. gaseous and injectable, with examples of each class and some of their given properties and adverse effects.
- Be able to discuss the blood:gas and oil:gas partition coefficients and the MAC with their relevance to general anaesthetics.
- Be able to give an account of the use of muscle relaxants with examples.

A definition of general anaesthesia

- State of unconsciousness and loss of pain appreciation due to the action of a chemical agent administered either by inhalation or by IV injection.

Before surgery

- Premedication aims and drugs used (not used as much as previously):
  - allay anxiety, e.g. lorazepam
  - reduce secretions, e.g. atropine (or glycopyrronium chloride during surgery)
  - gastric volume reduction and pH increase to prevent acid respiration, e.g. use of omeprazole (proton pump inhibitor) or ranitidine (H2-antagonist).

Aims of general anaesthesia

- Abolish the patient's awareness of the operational procedures.
- Abolish the sensation of pain during the operation.

The ideal general anaesthetic

- Is safe for the patient, e.g. wide margin between anaesthetic level (Stage 3) and toxic levels in the body (Stage 4).
- Is safe to administer, e.g. non-flammable.
- Rapidly brings the patient to Stage 3 of anaesthesia.
- Ensures that the patient feels no pain and does not respond to any external stimuli.
- Does not impair renal or cardiovascular function.
- Allows recovery without after-effects, e.g. hangover.

At present, no anaesthetic in use fulfils all these criteria fully.

Stages of general anaesthesia

- Stage 1: induction stage; period between start of drug administration and loss of consciousness.
- Stage 2: excitement stage; a dangerous stage best passed through rapidly, characterised by, for example, violent spontaneous movements of limbs, salivation (with dangers of asphyxiation), irregular respiration, exaggerated cough and retching reflexes.
- Stage 3: surgical anaesthesia; respiration becomes regular and with increasing build-up of anaesthetic may become shallow; cessation of spontaneous movement; some reflexes still present; muscle tone lessens until muscles relax.
- Stage 4: stage of medullary suppression; loss of respiration and cardiovascular collapse; death within minutes without respiratory and circulatory support.

Historical note: these stages were formulated based on the stages observed with the use of ether.

Types of general anaesthetics

- Administered by inhalation.
- Administered by IV injection.

General anaesthetics administered by inhalation

- May be gases or volatile liquids: desflurane, halothane, isoflurane, nitrous oxide, sevoflurane.

The blood:gas partition coefficient

- A measure of solubility of the anaesthetic in blood.
- The lower the blood:gas coefficient, the quicker the rate of onset and recovery.

The oil:gas partition coefficient

- A measure of solubility of the anaesthetic in fat.
- A measure of anaesthetic potency.

The minimum alveolar concentration (MAC)

- The concentration of the vapour in the lungs needed to prevent movement in 50% of subjects in response to a painful stimulus; a measure of potency.

TABLE 35.1 THE RELATIONSHIP BETWEEN MAC AND OIL:GAS PARTITION COEFFICIENT

ANAESTHETIC	MAC (%)	OIL:GAS PARTITION COEFFICIENT	MAIN ADVERSE EFFECTS AND DISADVANTAGES*
Nitrous oxide	100	1.4	Small anaemia risk
Desflurane	5	23	Bronchospasm
Isoflurane	2	91	Few: coronary ischaemia
Enflurane	1.4	98	Very rare: convulsions, malignant hyperthermia
Halothane	0.75	220	Hepatotoxicity with repeated use; dysrhythmias; hypotension
Methoxyflurane	0.16	930	Slow onset and recovery

Note: Strong correlation between MAC (potency) and oil:gas partition coefficient

General anaesthetics administered by injection

- Useful for induction of anaesthesia: etomidate, ketamine, midazolam, propofol, thiopentone sodium (thiopental).

TABLE 35.2 INTRAVENOUS ANAESTHETIC AGENTS

ANAESTHETIC	INDUCTION/RECOVERY SPEED	SOME ADVERSE EFFECTS AND DISADVANTAGES*
Etomidate	Fast/fast	Muscle movements
Ketamine**	Slow/variable	Vivid dreams during recovery
Midazolam	Onset slowest	Respiratory arrest with rapid injection
Propofol	Fast/very fast	Pain during injection; convulsions
Thiopental	Fast/slow	Cardio-respiratory depression

Note: most cause hypotension and apnoea during induction
*Not comprehensive (*see* BNF for more information)
**Rarely used in UK; ketamine is used as a racemic mixture or as separated enantiomers

Muscle relaxants

- Non-depolarising neuromuscular blocking drugs:

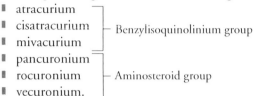

  - atracurium
  - cisatracurium — Benzylisoquinolinium group
  - mivacurium
  - pancuronium
  - rocuronium — Aminosteroid group
  - vecuronium.

Surgical use

- Relaxation of vocal cords to facilitate tracheal intubation.
- Relaxation of muscles during surgery, especially diaphragm and abdominal muscles.
- Atracurium can be used in patients with kidney or liver problems (non-enzymatic metabolism).
- Mivacurium contraindicated in patients deficient in cholinesterase.
- Histamine release to a greater or lesser extent with benzylisoquinolinium group except with cisatracurium.
- Rocuronium useful when fast onset required.
- Vecuronium low on cardiovascular adverse effects.

Depolarising neuromuscular blocking drugs

- Suxamethonium (synonyms: scoline; succinylcholine):
  - structurally, two molecules of ACh joined together
  - useful when short-acting effect wanted; fast onset and offset
  - action in two phases, initially stimulation resulting in fasciculations, followed by ACh receptor insensitivity to ACh and blockade
  - can cause malignant hyperthermia (rare but potentially fatal) and cardiac irregularities.

Clinical note: patients given muscle relaxants must be kept on assisted respiration until the muscle relaxant effect has been reversed.

Chapter 35 Quiz

ANSWER T (TRUE) OR F (FALSE)

1. Premedication is used to dry secretions and allay anxiety. ☐

2. Proton pump inhibitors may be used before surgery to reduce risk of acid respiration. ☐

3. General anaesthetics are administered by inhalation or injection. ☐

4. The ideal general anaesthetic:

    Has a narrow gap between Stages 3 and 4. ☐

    Is non-flammable if a gas. ☐

    Brings the patient slowly to Stage 3. ☐

    Does not impair cardiovascular or renal function. ☐

    Abolishes appreciation of pain during surgery. ☐

    Does not impair cardiovascular function. ☐

    Has no hangover or after-effects. ☐

5. There is a strong positive correlation between the MAC and the oil:gas partition coefficient. ☐

6. Halothane is associated with hepatotoxicity. ☐

7. Ketamine can cause nightmares during recovery. ☐

8. Thiopental can cause cardio-respiratory depression. ☐

9. Suxamethonium is a non-depolarising muscle relaxant. ☐

36 Parkinson's disease

Learning objectives
- Know what changes in the brain cause Parkinson's disease.
- Be aware of the consequences for the patient.
- Be able to list the main classes of drugs used to treat Parkinson's disease with examples.
- Know the use and adverse effects of levodopa.

Parkinson's disease introduction
- Incidence: usually ~ 65 years, may present earlier; no sexual bias.
- Is a degenerative disorder of the CNS resulting in:
  - impairment and loss of motor skills (for example):
    - bradykinesia (slowness of voluntary movements)
    - festination (stumbling, jerky fast gait usually ends in a fall)
    - hypokinesia (inhibition of voluntary movements)
    - akinesia (eventual loss of voluntary movements; 'gait freezing')
    - loss of postural reflexes and instability (patient falls)
    - tremor
    - rigidity
  - autonomic disturbances (for example):
    - constipation
    - gradual weight loss
    - hypotension and syncope (fainting)
    - nocturia (bedwetting)
  - disorders of the senses:
    - microsmia and anosmia (impairment and eventual loss of sense of smell)
    - double vision
  - speech disturbances
  - cognitive disturbances:
    - impaired short-term memory
    - progressive slowing of thought

- ◆ dysfunction of attention priorities
- ◆ eventual dementia
- ▌ sleep disorders:
  - ◆ nightmares, vivid dreams
  - ◆ daytime drowsiness
- ▌ mood disturbances:
  - ◆ depression
  - ◆ anxiety.

Aetiology of Parkinson's disease and symptoms

- ▓ Causative factors resulting in spontaneous onset unknown.
- ▓ Possible genetic factors.
- ▓ Drug-induced:
  - ▌ antipsychotics
  - ▌ MPTP ((1-methyl 4-phenyl 1,2,3,6-tetrahydropyridine), a contaminant of illicitly produced meperidine, an opioid analgesic.
- ▓ Possible environmental and personal history factors:
  - ▌ pesticides
  - ▌ metals, e.g. iron, manganese
  - ▌ previous trauma to head.

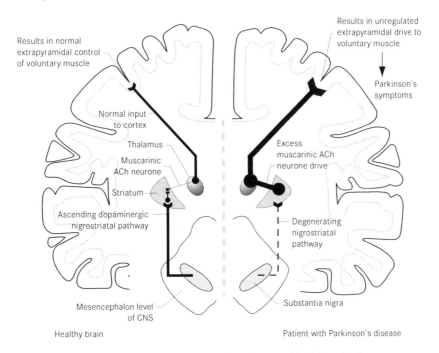

FIGURE 36.1 Central pathways involved in the aetiology of Parkinson's disease.

Neurological changes causing Parkinson's disease

- Progressive loss of the nigrostriatal dopaminergic pathway, resulting in;
- Reduced inhibitory dopaminergic inputs to the striatum, resulting in;
- Unregulated firing of the cholinergic extrapyramidal motor system of the brain, which normally controls fine voluntary movements, which in turn results in, tremor, loss of voluntary movement.

Terminology note: extrapyramidal refers to any of the brain structures affecting movement, excluding the motor neurons, the motor cortex, and the pyramidal tract, but including the corpus striatum, the substantia nigra and subthalamic nucleus, and connections with the midbrain.

Diagnosis of Parkinson's disease

- Patient's medical history.
- PET scan.

Treatment of Parkinson's disease with drugs

- Antimuscarinic drugs:
    - benzatropine mesilate
    - procyclidine hydrochloride   } Block muscarinic ACh receptors in the brain
    - trihexiphenidyl hydrochloride.
- Dopamine agonists:
    - apomorphine
    - bromocriptine
    - cabergoline
    - lisuride   } Agonists at dopamine D_2 receptors in the striatum
    - pergolide
    - pramipexole
    - rotigotine
    - ropinorole.
- Dopamine precursor (crosses blood–brain barrier; dopamine does not):
    - levodopa, which is converted in the brain to dopamine plus:
        - carbidopa, or   } Dopa-decarboxylase inhibitors: do not cross the blood–brain
        - benserazide   barrier; thus reducing *peripheral* adverse effects of dopamine
    - co-beneldopa: a mixture of benserazide and levodopa
    - co-careldopa: a mixture of carbidopa and levodopa.
- Monoamine oxidase –B (MAOI-B) inhibitors:
    - block the enzyme that breaks down dopamine at the synapse, thus prolonging its action; examples: rasagiline and selegiline.

- COMT inhibitors:
  - inhibit COMT (L-aromatic amino acid decarboxylase) which catalyses the conversion of dopa to dopamine (*see* p. 45), thereby allowing more levodopa to get into the brain; examples: entacapone and tolcapone.

Levodopa

- Still the most widely prescribed drug for Parkinson's disease, despite its adverse effects.
- Indication for use:
  - Parkinson's disease, but not for drug-induced parkinsonism.
- Preparations prescribed:
  - levodopa alone discontinued in BNF
  - co-beneldopa
    - capsules
    - modified release capsules
  - co-careldopa tablets
    - tablets
    - modified release tablets
    - with entacapone
    - intestinal gel using an enteral tube.

Adverse effects of levodopa

- Initial adverse effects when starting levodopa:
  - nausea
  - anorexia } Caused by peripheral conversion of levodopa to dopamine
  - central disturbances:
    - drowsiness
    - hallucinations
    - nightmares
    - headaches
    - 'sudden sleep' onset with levodopa/dopa decarboxylase preparations; dangerous if driving.
- Longer-term adverse effects with levodopa:
  - predictability and effectiveness become variable and unpredictable
  - 'on-off' phenomenon occurs; patient on levodopa suddenly 'freezes' when in the process of moving and cannot move
  - dyskinesia; the patient has involuntary writhing movements of limbs and face, and this is extremely unpleasant for the patient
  - 'end-of-dose' deterioration; the duration of benefit with levodopa becomes shorter and shorter with each dose
  - this can be dealt with by giving entacapone with the levodopa.

- Contraindications to levodopa include:
  - pregnancy
  - breast-feeding
  - closed-angle glaucoma.

Other treatments, inputs and research

- Family and supporting organisations.
- Regular physical exercises are recommended to help improve maintaining balance and muscle mobility and tone.
- In some patients brain surgery (for example):
  - pallidotomy (making surgical lesions in the globus pallidus)
  - lesions in the subthalamic nucleus
  - deep brain stimulation.
- Neuroprotective agents, e.g. drugs that are antiapoptotic (blocking programmed cell death).
- Transplantation of brain tissue; not successful at present.
- Gene therapy to boost inhibitory neurotransmitters, e.g. GABA; currently being researched.

Chapter 36 Quiz

ANSWER T (TRUE) OR F (FALSE)

1. Parkinson's disease:
   Is a degenerative disorder of the CNS. ☐
   Usually presents between 50–65 years. ☐
   Involves a progressive loss of sensory function. ☐
   Is caused by degeneration of CNS noradrenergic neurones. ☐ ☐
2. Parkinson's disease is caused by unregulated firing of the
   cholinergic extrapyramidal system of the brain. ☐
3. Drugs such MPTP can cause parkinsonian symptoms. ☐
4. Parkinson's disease is treated with:
   Antimuscarinic drugs. ☐
   Dopamine agonists. ☐
   Monoamine oxidase-B inhibitors. ☐
   COMT inhibitors. ☐
5. Co-beneldopa is a mixture of levodopa and carbidopa. ☐

6. Adverse effects of levodopa include:

   Nausea and vomiting initially. ☐

   Nightmares and hallucinations. ☐

   Headaches. ☐

   Dyskinesia. ☐

   'On-off' phenomenon. ☐

   Insomnia. ☐

7. Contraindications for levodopa include pregnancy, breast-feeding and closed-angle glaucoma. ☐

37 Epilepsy

Learning objectives

- Be able to describe what epilepsy is.
- Know the names of the main types of epilepsy.
- Be aware that certain drugs can cause epileptiform seizures and give some examples.
- Be aware of the given views and criteria whether or not an apparently first seizure requires subsequent drug treatment.
- Be ready to give:
  - a list of some drugs used to treat partial seizures and some of their reported adverse effects
  - a list of some drugs used to treat tonic-clonic seizures and some of their reported adverse effects.
- Know what is meant by status epilepticus and be able to describe the four stages of status epilepticus and the given information on how drugs are used to deal with it.

Epilepsy

- Is the occurrence of recurrent seizures.
- Seizures are transient, clinical manifestations of abnormally high and inappropriate stimulation of cortical neuronal circuits.
- Is a chronic medical condition.
- May:
  - have a known cause, e.g. brain damage through trauma
  - be idiopathic (unknown aetiology).
- Seizures may be:
  - partial, through discharges from focal cortical regions, usually in the amygdala or hippocampus, and may be:
    - simple
    - complex.
  - synchronous, through electrical discharges over both cerebral hemispheres; characterised by loss of consciousness and clonic and

tonic convulsions, followed by coma and gradual return to confused consciousness.

Nomenclature note: tonic means persistent contraction of the skeletal muscles; clonic means intermittent contractions and relaxing of skeletal muscle.

- absence (used to be called *petit mal*), suffered by children, and may be:
  - atypical: prolonged seizures usually caused by pre-existing neuronal damage, characterised by prolonged loss of contact with the child's environment
  - typical: less common, consisting of frequent, momentary loss of contact with the child's environment.

Theoretical considerations
- Epilepsy may be the result of an imbalance caused by neuronal damage to the normal counterinfluences of the inhibitory GABAergic and excitatory glutaminergic neurotransmitter systems in the brain.

Drug-induced seizures
- Drugs can cause epileptiform seizures – seizures resembling epileptic seizures (for example):
  - antidepressants, e.g. imipramine
  - antibiotics, e.g. isoniazid
  - CNS stimulants
  - endocrine-related drugs, e.g. insulin
  - general anaesthetics, e.g. halothane
  - cardioactive drugs, e.g. lidocaine.

Treatment of epilepsy with drugs
- No drug treatment for an isolated, one-off and apparently unprovoked seizure if:
  - there is no evidence of structural brain damage
  - there are no greatly abnormal EEG changes
  - the seizure can be put down to stress, prolonged insomnia or febrile conditions, for example.

Prescribing note: this is still a controversial area, and some authorities advocate drugs always after a first seizure to reduce the likelihood of another seizure.

- The primary aim is to prevent seizures.
- Some practitioners hold that drug treatment should initially consist of monotherapy.

Partial seizures – adverse effects

- Starting drugs include:
  - carbamazepine ⎤
  - lamotrigine ⎦—————
  - gabapentin (adjunct therapy) ⎤—
  - levetiracetam ⎤
  - oxcarbazepine ⎦ Neurological problems
  - tiagabine ⎦
  - sodium valproate ——— Weight gain, hair loss, tremor ⎤
  - topiramate. ———————— Sedation, kidney stone ⎦ Teratogen

Skin rashes, nausea, headaches, teratogenic; carbamazepine may cause double vision, lamotrigine insomnia; do NOT stop carbamazepine (or other drugs for epilepsy) suddenly as this can precipitate a seizure

Effects on liver function, weight gain

Precautionary note: these are all examples for study and are not comprehensive; Prescribers MUST obtain full patient histories and the advice of colleagues before prescribing.

Precautions and contraindications

- Sodium valproate:
  - associated with occasional fatal liver failure in young children
  - use with caution or not at all in patients with SLE or breast-feeding
  - contraindicated with: porphyria, active liver disease and family history of liver disease.
- Carbamazepine:
  - precaution if there is: a family history of adverse haematological reaction to drugs; a history of skin or liver problems
  - contraindicated with: porphyria, patients with atrio-ventricular conduction problems unless paced, family history of bone marrow depression.
- Lamotrigine:
  - monitor patients for liver and kidney function and clotting time.
- Topiramate:
  - may cause eye problems, especially raised intra-ocular pressure (danger of glaucoma)
  - ensure that patients on topiramate are adequately hydrated and that there is no history of patient or family kidney problems as topiramate is excreted mainly via the kidneys
  - contraindicated with: breast-feeding.
- Drugs contraindicated with absence seizures include:
  - phenobarbital
  - primidone
  - phenytoin.

Generalised (tonic-clonic) seizures

- Some general principles preventing seizures with drugs:
  - monotherapy at first preferable, but if not a combination may be needed
  - if drug is ineffective, the dose may need increasing
  - ensure patient is not also using previously prescribed anticonvulsants; check for all other medication use
  - be aware of patient compliance problems, especially elderly patients; regular monitoring of drug plasma concentrations may be needed
  - persistent drug failure may need family co-operation and counselling.
- Drugs used:
  - phenytoin; historically the mainstay but now supplanted in more affluent countries by other drugs, mainly because of pharmacokinetics and adverse effects (for example):
    - zero order kinetics, i.e. rate of metabolism and elimination is independent of plasma concentration; this means toxic concentrations are eliminated at the same rate as lower concentrations; dangerous for the patient
    - liver enzyme induction; results in accelerated metabolism of other drugs, e.g. OCs, thyroxine
    - strong plasma binding; phenytoin displaces other bound drugs, which can make them toxic, e.g. aspirin
    - gum hypertrophy, hirsutism and greasy skin
  - phenobarbital; historical interest, but largely discontinued in developed countries due to (for example):
    - sedative action
    - neurotoxicity
  - benzodiazepines
    - clobazam ⎤
    - clonazepam ⎬— Adverse effects include sedation; dependence and seizure-producing withdrawal symptoms
    - diazepam ⎦
  - lamotrigine
  - sodium valproate
  - carbamazepine
  - oxcarbazepine.

See NICE guidelines for treating epilepsy in adults and children: http://guidance.nice.org.uk/CG20.

Status epilepticus

- Is the persistent occurrence of a tonic-clonic seizure for more than 30 minutes.

- Should be assumed if a tonic-clonic seizure persists for more than 5 minutes and treated accordingly.
- Patients most at risk are:
  - children
  - mentally ill patients
  - patients with frontal lobe damage
  - dangers include ischaemia, hypoxia and brain damage through excess neuro-excitatory activity.
- Must be treated fast:
  - Stage 1 – within 10 minutes of seizure: secure airways, oxygen, cardiopulmonary resuscitation if needed
  - Stage 2 – within 30 minutes:
    - ventilation if respiratory failure
    - IV lines for fluid and anticonvulsant drugs (each drug at a different body site)
    - lorazepam or other benzodiazepine IV + glucose if hypoglycaemic
    - monitor ECG, biochemical parameters, haematological parameters, kidney and liver function.
  - Stage 3 – if patient not recovered by 30 minutes:
    - patient transferred to intensive care
    - drugs, e.g. IV loading dose of phenytoin or phosphenytoin or sub-anaesthetic dose of phenobarbital; followed by repeated oral or IV administration; alternatively, combination therapy with diazepam (fast onset) and phenytoin (prolonged action).
  - Stage 4 – after 60–90 minutes; refractory status epilepticus with a poor prognosis, high morbidity and mortality; treatment involves ventilation, IV propofol or thiopental and continuous midazolam IV.

Chapter 37 Quiz

ANSWER T (TRUE) OR F (FALSE)

1. Epilepsy:

    Is the occurrence of recurrent seizures. ☐

    Is sometimes due to brain damage through trauma. ☐

    May be idiopathic. ☐

    May involve imbalances in glutaminergic/GABAergic systems. ☐

    Can occur in children. ☐

    Is usually by cerebella damage. ☐

2. Absence seizures may be typical or atypical. ☐

3. Atypical seizures are prolonged. ☐

4. Atypical seizures are usually caused by pre-existing neuronal damage. ☐

5. Typical seizures are frequent, momentary episodes. ☐

6. Drug treatment *may* be inappropriate if:

   There are no abnormal EEG changes. ☐

   The patient had prolonged insomnia. ☐

   There is no evidence of structural brain damage. ☐

   The patient has a fever. ☐

7. The primary aim of drug therapy is to revive the patient. ☐

8. Starting drugs for partial seizures include carbamazepine. ☐

9. Gabapentin may be added as an adjunct drug for partial seizures. ☐

10. Sodium valproate and topiramate have a risk of being teratogenic. ☐

11. A family history of bone marrow depression is a contraindication for carbamazepine. ☐

12. Patients on topiramate must be adequately hydrated. ☐

13. General principles for drug treatment for generalised seizures include:

    Multiple drugs at first. ☐

    Increasing dose of first drug if ineffective. ☐

    Adequate supervision of patient compliance. ☐

    Monitoring for adverse effects, e.g. regular blood tests. ☐

14. Phenytoin has the following disadvantages:

    First order kinetics. ☐

    High plasma protein binding. ☐

    Many drug interactions through, e.g. enzyme liver induction. ☐

    Adverse effects, e.g. gum hypertrophy. ☐

15. Benzodiazepines are not associated with severe withdrawal problems. ☐

38 Alzheimer's disease

Learning objectives ■ Alzheimer's disease ■ Stages of Alzheimer's disease for treatment purposes ■ Drugs used

Learning objectives

■ Know that Alzheimer's disease is an age-related degenerative brain disease.
■ Be aware of the β-amyloid plaque implication in the aetiology of the disease.
■ Be able to list the stages and drugs currently used.

Alzheimer's disease

■ Is a neurodegenerative disease in the cortical areas of the brain.
■ Is anecdotally linked to increased longevity.
■ Cause unknown, but possession of the Apo-E4 allele may predispose carriers to a risk.
■ Involves:
   ▮ disruption of normal cortical organisation, probably through deposition of β-amyloid protein plaques, and
   ▮ formation of neurofibrillary tangles
   ▮ possible disruption of cholinergic pathways (*see* below).
■ Results in:
   ▮ progressive loss of cognitive function, involving loss of:
      ♦ attention
      ♦ disorientation (in later stages)
      ♦ language usage
      ♦ memory
      ♦ problem solving ability.

Stages of Alzheimer's disease for treatment purposes

■ Stage 1: mild-moderate.
■ Stage 2: moderate-severe. ⎦ Assessed partly using MMSE (Mini-mental state examination)

Drugs used

■ Mild-moderate (mainly):
   ▮ donezepil
   ▮ galantamine ⎬ Reversible acetylcholinesterase inhibitors; inhibit ACh breakdown
   ▮ rivastigmine.

- Moderate-severe:
  - memantine; non-competitive antagonist at:
    - central nicotinic ACh receptors
    - 5-HT3 receptors
    - glutamatergic NMDA receptors.

Clinical note: The use of memantine is controversial and at time of writing is not recommended for moderate to severe Alzheimer's disease by NICE in the UK.

- Administration of drugs:
  - orally as tablets (donezepil and galantamine, or as capsules rivastigmine).
- Adverse effects reflect parasympathomimetic actions and include:
  - nausea, vomiting, diarrhoea
  - psychiatric disturbances
  - anorexia
  - headache
  - dizziness
  - rhinitis
  - diarrhoea.
- Contraindications for all these parasympathomimetic drugs include:
  - breast-feeding
  - pregnancy
  - Parkinson's disease.

39 Antidepressant drugs

Learning objectives ■ Features of clinical depression ■ Monoamine theory of depression ■ Antidepressant drugs ■ SSRIs ■ Monoamine oxidase inhibitors (MAOIs) ■ Tricyclic and tetracyclic antidepressants

Learning objectives

- Be able to give some features of clinical depression.
- Be able to list the major classes of antidepressants currently used.
- Know what is meant by the monoamine theory of depression.
- Be able to give examples of drugs used within the three main classes of antidepressants and have some knowledge of their major adverse effects and contraindications.

Features of clinical depression

- Low energy.
- Low sense of self-worth.
- Low libido.
- Low mood.
- Loss of enjoyment.
- Lethargy.
- Suicide risk.
- Often anxiety and insomnia, waking very early.
- Panic attacks.

Monoamine theory of depression

- Abnormal central monoamine neurotransmitter function involving norepinephrine and serotonergic systems may be responsible for depression, but the mechanisms involved are unknown with certainty.

Antidepressant drugs

- Monoamine oxidase inhibitors.
- Tricyclic antidepressants.]—— Largely historical now; superseded by:
- SSRIs.

SSRIs

- Mechanism of action: prolong endogenous 5-HT neurotransmitter activity in the brain by blocking re-uptake into the presynaptic nerve terminal.
- Examples include:
  - citalopram
  - escitalopram
  - fluoxetine
  - fluvoxamine
  - paroxetine
  - sertraline.
- Formulation:
  - oral tablets or capsules
  - oral drops.
- Adverse effects (not comprehensive):
  - suicide risk (*see* also below)
  - withdrawal symptoms if abruptly stopped
  - GIT:
    - nausea, vomiting
    - diarrhoea, constipation, abdominal cramps
  - appetite stimulant and weight gain
  - movement problems, e.g. dyskinesia
  - hypersensitivity reactions:
    - angioedema
    - photosensitivity
    - urticaria
    - risk of anaphylaxis.
- Precautions and contraindications include:
  - do not prescribe during the manic phase
  - diabetes
  - poorly controlled epilepsy ⎤
  - cardiovascular problems   ⎬ Patients need regular and frequent monitoring if on SSRIs
  - closed-angle glaucoma   ⎦
  - risk of suicide in adolescents and young adults – best avoided.

Monoamine oxidase inhibitors (MAOIs)

- Safety note: not used much any more, especially because of their interaction with dietary tyramine in cheese and wine, which promotes norepinephrine (NE) release from the nerve terminal. MAOIs block NE breakdown, which causes a potentially fatal hypertensive crisis.
- Mechanism of action: blocks the breakdown of norepinephrine after release as a neurotransmitter, thus potentiating its action.

- Examples include:
  - phenelzine
  - isocarbazid
  - tranylcypromine
  - meclobamide – reversible and therefore safer.

Irreversible – block MAOI activity for days to weeks

Mechanism note: MAOI exists in two forms MAOI-A and MAOI-B; anti-depressants mentioned above block mainly MAOI-A.

Tricyclic and tetracyclic antidepressants

- Examples include:
  - amitriptyline
  - doselepin HCl
  - imipramine HCl
  - mianserin (tetracyclic)
  - nortriptylene
  - clomipramine
  - doxepin
  - lofepramine
  - mirtazepine (tetracyclic)
  - trimipramine.

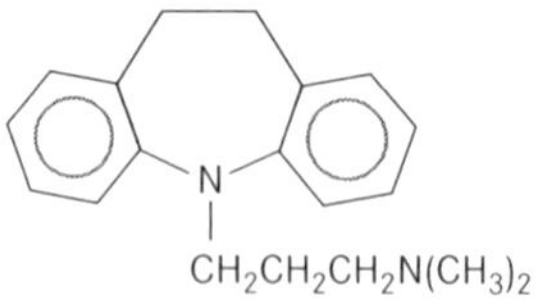

Imipramine (tricyclic)

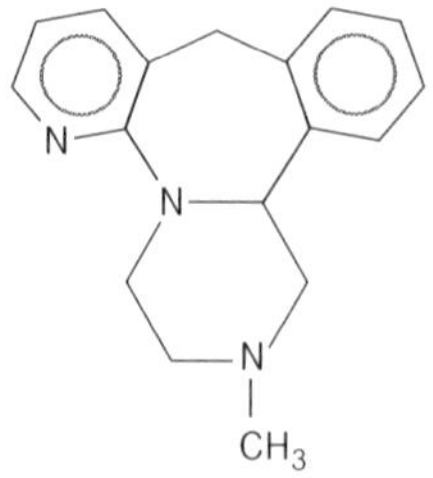

$CH_2CH_2CH_2N(CH_3)_2$

Mirtazepine (tetracyclic)

CH_3

FIGURE 39.1 Structures of imipramine and mirtazepine.

- Mechanisms of action: generally, inhibition of norepinephrine and 5-HT re-uptake into the presynaptic nerve terminal (*see* Figure 39.2); some e.g. imipramine, have significant dopamine D_1 and D_2 receptor blocking activity.
- Indications:
  - moderate/severe depression with sleep and appetite disturbances
  - panic attacks
  - some, e.g. doxepin and trimipramine, are also sedative.
- Uses, adverse effects, precautions and contraindications:
  - long delay before benefit seen (may be 2–3 weeks)
  - ECT (electroconvulsant) therapy may be needed initially
  - many adverse effects due to widespread interference with adrenergic and serotonergic activity centrally and peripherally (for example):
    - dry mouth, postural hypotension, tachycardia, behavioural

disturbances, e.g. paranoia, delirium in children (*see* BNF for more comprehensive details)

- precautions include:
  - cardiac problems
  - thyroid disease
  - breast-feeding and pregnancy
  - anaesthesia
- contraindications include:
  - arrhythmias
  - recent myocardial infarction
  - heart block
  - patients in manic phase
  - hepatic disease.
- Other antidepressants:
  - trazodone
    - neither tri-nor tetracyclic
    - mechanism: 5-HT re-uptake inhibitor + blockade of 5-HT$_2$ receptors.

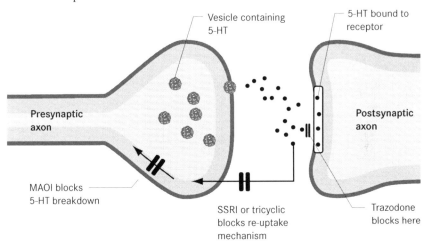

FIGURE 39.2 Mechanism of action of SSRIs, tricyclic antidepressants and trazodone.

Chapter 39 Quiz

ANSWER T (TRUE) OR F (FALSE)

1. Depression may be caused by low monoaminergic brain activity. ☐
2. MAOIs are the main drugs used to treat depression. ☐
3. SSRIs:

    Prolong brain 5-HT activity by blocking re-uptake of 5-HT. ☐

    Include citalopram. ☐

    In young people may pose a suicide risk. ☐

    Are useful in the manic phase. ☐
4. Precautions for SSRIs include:

    Diabetes. ☐

    Epilepsy. ☐

    Closed angle glaucoma. ☐
5. Adverse effects of SSRIs include:

    Withdrawal symptoms. ☐

    Diarrhoea. ☐

    Weight gain ☐

    Abdominal cramps. ☐

    Hypersensitivity reactions. ☐
6. MAOIs:

    Are the mainstay of treatment for depression. ☐

    Include isocarbazid. ☐

    Are very dangerous with wine or cheese. ☐
7. Tricyclic antidepressants inhibit re-uptake of 5-HT and NE. ☐
8. Trimipramine is a tricyclic antidepressant. ☐
9. Tricyclic antidepressants block acetylcholine reuptake. ☐
10. Tricyclics are not recommended for panic attacks. ☐
11. Tricyclics are indicated for moderate to severe depression with sleep disturbances. ☐
12. ECT therapy may be needed initially when using tricyclics. ☐
13. Tricyclics can cause paranoia as an adverse effect. ☐
14. Tricyclics are contraindicated after a recent myocardial infarction. ☐
15. Trazodone works by blocking MAO. ☐

40 Anxiolytic drugs

Learning objectives ■ Clinical anxiety ■ Treatment ■ Treatment with drugs ■
Benzodiazepines ■ Patient compliance

Learning objectives

- Know what is meant by clinical anxiety.
- Be aware of some of the symptoms and of the various non-drug treatments.
- Know the classes of drugs mentioned here for treatment with examples and adverse effects, particularly the withdrawal problems with benzodiazepines.

Clinical anxiety

- Is the chronic occurrence of sensations of fear and apprehension.
- Is not a 'one-off' occurrence but can increase in intensity and become debilitating.
- Is often irrational.
- Has been variously classified as:
  - general anxiety
  - phobias
  - panic disorder
  - post-traumatic stress disorder
  - obsessive compulsive disorder
  - generalised anxiety disorder (GAD).
- May present with symptoms including:
  - insomnia
  - depression
  - pessimism
  - hypochondria
  - loss of libido
  - GIT upsets and frequent urination
  - headache
  - tachycardia
  - panic.

Treatment

- Counselling.
- Support groups.
- Cognitive behavioural therapy. ⎤
- Self-help including exercise.   ├── Beyond the scope of this book
- Drugs.   ⎦

Treatment with drugs

- SSRIs:
  - fluoxetine
  - paroxetine.
- Benzodiazepines:
  - diazepam
  - lorazepam
  - oxazepam.

Benzodiazepines

- Are associated with:
  - dependence
  - severe withdrawal problems
  - paradoxical aggressive behaviour
  - amnesia, ataxia and syncope in elderly patients.
- Should not be prescribed for more than four weeks.
- Are contraindicated in:
  - panic attacks
  - sleep apnoea syndrome
  - acute pulmonary insufficiency
  - respiratory depression
  - severe liver problems.

Patient compliance

- Is generally a problem with patients suffering with anxiety and depression.
- Is often compromised by:
  - delayed onset of drug action
  - adverse effects of drugs, e.g. paranoia
  - patient's reluctance to take the drug, e.g. through paranoia.

Chapter 40 Quiz

ANSWER T (TRUE) OR F (FALSE)

1. Clinical anxiety:

   Is characterised mainly by depression. ☐

   Is a recurring problem for the patient. ☐

   May bring on panic attacks. ☐

   Symptoms include:

   Insomnia. ☐

   Pessimism. ☐

   Euphoria. ☐

   Loss of libido. ☐

   Hypochondria. ☐

2. Drugs used include SSRIs. ☐

3. Benzodiazepines are associated with severe withdrawal symptoms. ☐

4. In elderly patients, benzodiazepines can produce amnesia and ataxia. ☐

5. Benzodiazepines should not be prescribed for more than 4 months. ☐

6. Benzodiazepines are contraindicated with:

   Panic attacks. ☐

   Sleep apnoea syndrome. ☐

   Acute pulmonary insufficiency. ☐

7. Compliance with drug regimes among anxious patients is often compromised because of adverse drug effects. ☐

41 Anti-infective drugs (antibiotics)

Learning objectives ■ Anti-infective agents ■ Antibacterial drugs ■ Bacterial resistance ■ Antiviral drugs ■ Antifungal drugs ■ Antiprotozoal drugs

Learning objectives
- Know what is meant by gram-negative and gram-positive.
- Know the difference between bacteriostatic and bactericidal.
- Be able to give some of the different classes of antibacterials with examples of drugs.
- Know the important factors determining choice of an antibacterial.
- Be able to give an account of bacterial resistance.
- Know some of the uses of antiviral, antifungal and antiprotozoal drugs and give examples.

Anti-infective agents
- Antibacterial drugs.
- Antifungal drugs.
- Antiviral drugs.
- Antiprotozoan drugs.

Antibacterial drugs
- Gram-negative. ⎤
- Gram-positive. ⎦ Based on bacterial cell wall colour with the gram stain (crystal violet); gram-positive turns violet/blue; gram negative turns red/pink
- Bacteriostatic – stop bacterial multiplication but do not kill.
- Bactericidal – kill the bacteria.
- Narrow spectrum – affect only gram-positive or gram-negative bacteria.
- Broad spectrum – affect a wide range of bacteria.
- Can be classified as (not comprehensive):
    - cephalosporins, e.g. cefaclor, cefadroxil, cefoxatime
    - penicillins, e.g. amoxicillin, benzyl penicillin, flucloxacillin, ticarcillin
    - macrolides, e.g. erythromycin, clarithromycin, clindamycin
    - aminoglycosides, e.g. gentamycin, neomycin, streptomycin, tobramycin
    - sulphonamides, e.g. co-trimoxazole, sulfadiazine, trimethoprim
    - polymyxins, e.g. colistin

▪ quinolones, e.g. ciprofloxacin
▪ rifamycins, e.g. rifampicin.

Choice of antibacterial drug depends on:

▪ Patient status, e.g. allergies, including allergies to drugs, kidney and liver function, age, ethnicity, degree of immunocompetence, route of administration, if female whether pregnant or breast-feeding.
▪ Nature of infective agent, e.g. identification of bacterial infection, tests for resistance to drugs.
▪ The site of infection and cellular or subcellular target (*see* Figure 41.1).

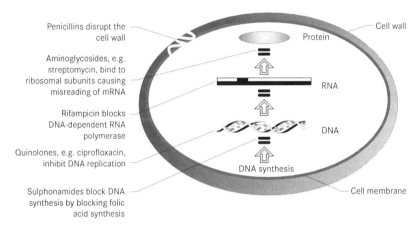

FIGURE 41.1 Mechanisms of action of antibiotics.

Bacterial resistance

▪ Is the failure of a drug to harm the infective organism (usually a bacterial cell line).
▪ May be caused by:
  ▪ incorrect use of drug, e.g. stopping treatment before course is run
  ▪ over-prescribing
  ▪ use of antibiotics in livestock
  ▪ incorrect diagnosis
  ▪ survival of mutant, resistant bacterial strains and their replication in the host.
▪ Underlying mechanisms include:
  ▪ bacterial degradation of the antibiotic, e.g. penicillins
  ▪ reduced ability of drug to penetrate the bacterial cell wall
  ▪ bacterial mutation to utilise folic acid without having to synthesis it
  ▪ mutation of bacterial cell wall penicillin-binding proteins (as happens with MRSA (methicillin-resistant *Staphylococcus aureus*).

Antiviral drugs (does not include vaccines)

- Are used mainly to treat HIV and herpes virus infections.
- Are used mainly in immunocompromised patients since many viral infections resolve without need for treatment in immunocompetent patients.
- Are used also for Herpes simplex (cold sores) and Varicella-zoster (virus causing chicken pox and shingles).
- Include aciclovir:
  - for systemic treatment of Herpes and Varicella, but does not eradicate these
  - which inhibits viral DNA polymerase.
- For HIV, include:
  - nucleoside reverse transcriptase inhibitors, e.g. abavacir
  - protease inhibitors, e.g. amprenavir
  - non-nucleoside reverse transcriptase inhibitors, e.g. efavirenz.

Antifungal drugs

- Are used to treat (for example):
  - aspergillosis (fungal growth, mainly in the respiratory tracts)
  - candidiasis ('thrush')
  - histoplasmosis (another lung-loving fungus, also called Darling's disease)
  - tinea (scalp ('ringworm'), and skin and nails)
- Include:
  - amphotericin
  - caspofungin
  - fluconazole
  - posaconazole
  - terbinafine.

Antiprotozoal drugs

- Antimalarial drugs:
  - treatment: artemether (semi-synthetic derivative of a Chinese medicine herb) with lumefantrine (benflumetol) for treating drug resistant strains of malaria caused by *Plasmodium falciparum*
  - prophylaxis: chloroquine, mefloquine, primaquine, proguanil HCl, for example.
- Amoebicides for entamoeba infections, e.g. amoebic dysentery:
  - diloxanide furoate, metronidazole, tinidazole.
- *Giardia lamblia*:
  - mepacrine HCl.
- Leishmaniasis from, e.g. sandfly bites, cutaneous boils; or dangerous if organism migrates into the viscera:

- amphotericin
- sodium stiboglutonate
- pentamidine isetionate.
- Toxoplasmosis (mainly in cats but transmissible to humans):
  - treatment often not required, but is if eyes are involved
  - pyrimethamine + sulphadiazine
  - pregnancy may pose problems for the foetus; spiramycin may be prescribed.

Chapter 41 Quiz

ANSWER T (TRUE) OR F (FALSE)

1. Gram-negative bacteria stain red with crystal violet. ☐
2. Bacteriostatic drugs do not kill the bacteria. ☐
3. Antibacterial drugs include:
   Cephalosporins. ☐
   Penicillins. ☐
   Aminoglycosides. ☐
   Sulphonamides. ☐
   Macrolides. ☐
4. The choice of an antibacterial depends on:
   The status of the patient. ☐
   The site of the infection. ☐
   The nature of the infective agent. ☐
   The cellular or subcellular target. ☐
   The patient's mental state. ☐
5. Bacterial resistance is failure of the drug to harm the infective organism. ☐
6. Bacterial resistance is caused by:
   The patient's immune system. ☐
   Incorrect use of the antibiotic. ☐
   Feeding antibiotics to livestock. ☐
   Incorrect diagnosis of the infecting organism. ☐
   Over-prescribing. ☐
7. Bacterial adaptations to antibiotics include:
   Increased capacity to degrade the antibiotic. ☐

Modification of the cell wall to exclude the drug. ☐

Cell wall mutation so the drug can't bind to it. ☐

Production of antibodies to the drug. ☐

8. Antiviral drugs:

Are used mainly for HIV and herpes. ☐

Include nucleoside reverse transcriptase inhibitors. ☐

9. Histoplasmosis is treated with abavacir. ☐

10. Antifungal drugs include fluconazole. ☐

11. Artemether is used as prophylaxis in malaria. ☐

12. Primaquine is prophylactic for malaria. ☐

13. Amoebic dysentery can be treated with metronidazole. ☐

14. Sand fly bites can cause Leishmaniasis. ☐

15. Leishmaniasis is treated with sodium stibogluconate. ☐

42 Chemotherapy for malignancy (cancer)

Learning objectives ■ Cancer chemotherapy ■ Mini glossary ■ Classes of drugs currently used for chemotherapy ■ Alkylating agents ■ Antimetabolites ■ Topoisomerase inhibitors ■ Antibiotics ■ Hormones and analogues ■ Breast cancer ■ Estrogens ■ Progestogens ■ Hormone antagonists and aromatase inhibitors ■ Prostate cancer ■ Monoclonal antibodies

Learning objectives

- Know the heading names for the classes of drugs given.
- Be able to give examples of drugs listed in all the categories listed.
- Know important disadvantages and adverse effects of alkylating agents.
- Know what is meant by antimetabolites and topoisomerase inhibitors.
- Be able to give a brief account of hormone analogues and antagonists in the treatment of cancer.
- Be able to give examples of monoclonal antibodies and their uses to treat cancer.

Cancer chemotherapy

- Is the use of chemicals to stop the growth of cancer cells and if possible kill them.
- These drugs are also referred to as 'cytotoxic', which means poisonous to cells.

Mini glossary

Adenocarcinoma: malignant epithelial cancer arising in glandular tissue, or one which has a glandular appearance and function, e.g. secretions.

Alkylation: adding alkyl groups, e.g. CH_3 or C_6H_{14} etc to other molecules

Carcinoma: cancer arising in epithelial tissue.

Chemotherapy: with respect to cancer treatment, refers specifically to cytotoxic drugs.

Cytotoxic: able to destroy cells; refers to drugs and to radiotherapy.

Indolent: slow-growing.

Isoprenoids: chemicals with a structure related to those of terpenoid hydro-carbons (corals produce these for self-defence).

Malignant: invasive, destructive cells, capable of proliferation in the body and potentially lethal.

Metastasis: spread of malignant tumour to other tissues in the body.

Mitosis: cell division with two daughter cells arising from one parent cell.

Radionuclide: chemical possessing a radioactive, particle-emitting nucleus, often used in nuclear medicine as a diagnostic tracer, e.g. ^{60}Cobalt, ^{90}Strontium.

Radiotherapy: treatment to kill cancer cells with penetrating radiation, e.g. X-rays or gamma rays.

Topoisomerase inhibitors: enzymes which affect the super-coiling of double-stranded DNA.

Tumour: abnormal swelling in or on the body.

Classes of drugs currently used for chemotherapy
- Alkylating agents.
- Antimetabolites.
- Topoisomerase inhibitors.
- Antibiotics which attack tumours.
- Hormones and analogues.
- Monoclonal antibodies (biological [US biologic] agents).

Terminology note: 'cytotoxic' here refers to a treatment that kills cells.

Historical note: alkylating agents were first developed as weapons of war.

Alkylating agents (not comprehensive)
- Bisulfan.
- Cyclophosphamide.
- Ifosfamide.
- Melphalan.
- Treosulphan.
- Carmustine.
- Estramustine.
- Lomustine.
- Thiotepa.

Actions and adverse effects of alkylating agents
- Cytotoxic; kill dividing cells.
- Non-selective; will also kill fast-dividing cells, for example:
  - gut epithelial cells ⟶ nausea, vomiting
  - hair follicles ⟶ hair loss (alopecia)
  - bone marrow ⟶ bone marrow depression
  - cells of the immune system ⟶ immunosuppressant
  - reproductive cells ⟶ teratogenic

Antimetabolites
- Block cell division by:
  - intercalating into new nuclear DNA or RNA
  - blocking cellular enzymes.

- Examples include:
  - capecitabine
  - cytarabine
  - fludarabine
  - gemcitabine
  - methotrexate.
  - cladribine
  - clofarabine
  - fluorouracil
  - mercaptopurine

Adverse actions

- Many for this group.
- Include myelosuppression (suppression of bone marrow blood cell production), nausea, vomiting, and mucositis (inflammation of GIT mucosal linings anywhere in the tract; often present as mouth ulcers).

Topoisomerase inhibitors

- Drugs that interfere with the normal supercoiling of DNA and with DNA replication and transcription; some are derived from plant alkaloids, e.g. *Podophyllum peltatum* (etoposide).
- Include:
  - amsacrine
  - topotecan
  - irinotecan
  - etoposide.

Antibiotics

- Include:
  - bleomycin
  - doxorubicin
  - idarubicin
  - mitoxantrone.
  - dactinomycin
  - epirubicin
  - mitomycin
- Act through a variety of actions, e.g. through generation of free radicals (e.g. mitomycin) or through actions on topoisomerase enzymes (e.g. doxorubicin).

Hormones and analogues

BREAST CANCER

- Estrogens.
- Hormone antagonist drugs.
- Progestogens.
- GnRH analogues.

ESTROGENS

- Ethinylestradiol for prostate cancer.
- Stilboestrol (an antiestrogen not much used now) for post-menopausal breast cancer.

PROGESTOGENS
- Medroxyprogesterone acetate in endometrial cancer.

Hormone antagonists and aromatase inhibitors
- Antiestrogens block the estrogen receptor:
  - tamoxifen: used in estrogen receptor-positive breast cancer
  - fulvestrant: post-menopausal women, if tamoxifen does not work.
- SERMs (selective estrogen receptor modulators):
  - toremifene for post-menopausal women with estrogen-responsive metastatic breast cancer.
- Aromatase inhibitors (the aromatase enzyme system normally converts androgen to estrogen); used in post-menopausal women only:
  - anastrozole ⎤
  - letrozole ⎦ — Non-steroidal
  - exemestane (steroidal).

Clinical note: breast cancers are graded as 1, 2 or 3; 1 being the most indolent (slow-growing), and after surgical removal the patient is often treated with hormonal therapy, for example tamoxifen (if estrogen receptor positive) and also with radiotherapy; a grade 3 tumour demands more aggressive chemotherapy with, for example, antibiotics or antimetabolites and radiotherapy.

PROSTATE CANCER
- Gonadotrophin releasing hormone (GnRH) analogues:
  - desensitises the anterior pituitary gland to GnRH, producing a reversible chemical castration to remove testosterone from the circulation
  - include:
    - bicalutamide
    - buserelin
    - goserelin
    - leuprorelin
    - triptorelin.

Cautionary note: with GnRH analogues, there is a risk, especially with initial use, of 'tumour flare', caused by the initial stimulant effect of GnRH analogues on testosterone production; it should be possible to reduce this risk by treating patients for whom a GnRH analogue has been prescribed with a testosterone receptor blocker, e.g. cyproterone acetate.

Monoclonal antibodies

- Are made using recombinant DNA technology.
- Target the body's own antigens which have been identified as mediating the neoplastic reaction (for example):
  - bevacizumab (MAB = monoclonal antibody)
    - blocks formation of new blood vessels, thus stopping blood supplies to the growing tumour
  - cetuximab
    - blocks the epidermal growth factor receptor; used for cell carcinoma of head and neck; colorectal cancer
  - rituximab
    - is a chimaeric (components from more than one species in the molecule) monoclonal antibody directed against CD20, which is a protein expressed on the surface of all mature B-cells and has no known ligand, but occurs on cells in: chronic lymphocytic leukemia, hairy cell leukaemia, lymphomas
  - trastuzumab (Herceptin)
    - is used to treat HER2-positive metastatic breast cancer
    - is a humanized monoclonal antibody that blocks the HER2/neu (erbB2) receptor by binding to the extracellular segment of the receptor
  - this results in the cell going into arrest in the G1 phase of the cell cycle, and further growth is stopped.

Chapter 42 Quiz

ANSWER T (TRUE) OR F (FALSE)

1. Cytotoxic means poisonous to cells. ☐
2. Alkylating agents are highly specific in targeting cancer cells. ☐
3. Adverse effects of alkylating agents include:
   Alopecia. ☐
   Teratogenicity. ☐
   Dementia. ☐
   GIT disturbances. ☐
   Bone marrow depression. ☐
4. Adverse effects of antimetabolites include:
   Myelosuppression. ☐

Mucositis. □

Nausea and vomiting. □

5. Topoisomerase inhibitors stimulate DNA supercoiling. □

6. Antibiotics:

May act through the generation of free radicals. □

May act on enzymes. □

7. Estrogens exacerbate breast cancer. □

8. Antiestrogens block estrogen action. □

9. Tamoxifen is used for estrogen receptor-positive malignancy. □

10. Toremifene is indicated for premenopausal women. □

11. Bevacizumab is a monoclonal antibody stimulating blood vessel growth (angiogenesis). □

12. Trastuzumab (Herceptin) is used for HER2-positive metastatic breast cancer. □

Quiz answers

Chapter 3 Quiz answers

T = TRUE   F = FALSE

1. Subcutaneous injection gives the most rapid onset of drug action.   F
   IV injection gives the most rapid onset.
2. Uncharged molecules are absorbed more rapidly after oral
   administration.   T
3. Drug distribution is independent of its lipid solubility.   F
   Lipid solubil ity *is* important for drug distribution in the body.
4. The higher the volume of distribution, the higher the dose that may be
   needed.   T
5. The plasma protein-bound drug is the form available to the tissues.   F
   The *free* drug in plasma is available to the tissues.
6. The major site of drug metabolism is the liver.   T
7. First pass metabolism can reduce the efficacy of a drug.   T
8. Phase I reactions conjugate the drug to (e.g.) a glucuronide.   F
   Phase II reactions conjugate the drug.
9. Metabolism is the invariable method for inactivating drugs.   F
   Some drugs are *activated* after metabolism.
10. Drugs are easier for the body to excrete when rendered more soluble.   T
11. Genetic factors can affect the degree of drug metabolism.   T
12. Most drugs are excreted via the faeces.   F
    Most drugs currently used are excreted via the kidneys.
13. Measurement of drug half-life is not used to measure the rate of drug
    excretion.   F
    Half-life *is* a measurement of drug excretion.
14. First order kinetics means that the rate of drug excretion is faster when
    plasma concentrations of the drug are higher.   T

Chapter 4 Quiz answers

T = TRUE   F = FALSE

1. Pharmacodynamics:
    Is the study of how the body processes the drug.   F
       It is the study of how the drug affects the body.
    Includes the study of receptor dynamics.   T
    Attempts to explain the cell's response to the drug.   T
2. The receptor:
    Is the cell's mechanism for recognising the drug.   T
    Is always situated on the membrane of the cell.   F
       May be intracellular, for example, steroid receptors.
    Has properties of high affinity binding and selectivity.   T
    Can bind only one ligand.   F
       Receptors can often bind more than one ligand.
3. The dose-response curve:
    Describes the relationship between dose and tissue response.   T
    Is useful because it has a linear segment.   F
       The $\log_{10}$ dose-response curve has a linear segment.
    Gives an approximate idea of the potency of a drug.   T
    Gives the drug dose above which there is no further increase in
    response.   T
4. The $\log_{10}$ dose-response curve:
    Can be used to compare drug potencies for a given parameter.   T
    Can be used to measure the potency of a drug antagonist.   T
5. An agonist is a drug that produces a response similar to that produced
    by an endogenous mediator.   T
6. An antagonist:
    Blocks the action of an agonist.   T
    May act by:
       a. Interfering with the metabolism of the agonist.   F
       b. Competing with the agonist at its receptor site.   T
       c. Blocking an ion channel in the cell membrane.   T
       d. Blocking downstream events e.g. transcription.   T
7. An antagonist's action:
    Cannot be reversed.   F
    May be competitive and reversible.   T
    May be irreversible and non-competitive.   T

Chapter 6 Quiz answers

T = TRUE   F = FALSE

1. The receptor:
   Is a protein able to recognise only one ligand.   F
     Can bind more than one ligand but is selective.
   Binds ligands with high affinity and selectivity.   T
   May be part of the cell membrane or occur intracellularly.   T
   Is the first step in the cell's recognition of extracellular ligands.   T
2. Ligand-gated ion channels:
   Consist of a ligand-binding site linked to an ion pore.   T
   Mediate long-delay transduction.   F
     Mediate *very short* delay transduction.
   Control ATP-gated channels.   T
   Mediate muscarinic ACh cellular responses.   F
     Mediate *nicotinic* ACh cellular responses.
3. Metabotropic receptors:
   Span cell membranes with 7 transmembrane domains.   T
   Have intracellular NH_2 terminals.   F
     Have *extracellular* NH_2 terminals.
   May activate intracellular second messenger systems.   T
   Include the insulin receptor.   T
4. Second messengers:
   Are so-called because they initiate intracellular responses to drugs.   T
   Are a means of amplifying cellular responses to a single drug molecule.   T
   Include cyclic AMP and diacylglycerol.   T

Chapter 7 Quiz answers

T = TRUE   F = FALSE

1. The autonomic nervous system controls voluntary movement.   F
     The autonomic nervous system is considered to be outside
   conscious control.
2. The ANS consists of sympathetic and parasympathetic divisions.   T
3. Afferent preganglionic fibres carry impulses to the target organs.   F
     Efferent postganglionic fibres carry impulses to the target organs.
4. Efferent parasympathetic, preganglionic fibres are generally long.   T
5. Afferent nerve fibres carry impulses from the CNS to the periphery.   F
     Afferent nerve fibres carry impulses from the periphery to the CNS.
6. ACh is released from presynaptic, preganglionic fibres in the ganglia.   T

7. ACh binds to postsynaptic nicotinic receptors in the ganglia.   T
8. ACh binds to postganglionic, postsynaptic adrenoceptors on target   F
   organs.
       ACh binds to postganglionic, postsynaptic *muscarinic receptors* on
   target organs.
9. Epinephrine is the major postganglionic neurotransmitter of the   F
   sympathetic division of the ANS.
       Norepinephrine is the major postganglionic neurotransmitter of the
   sympathetic division of the ANS.

Chapter 8 Quiz answers

T = TRUE   F = FALSE

1. The PNS is not essential for life.   F
       The PNS is essential for life maintenance.
2. PNS efferent outflows are via craniosacral regions.   T
3. The PNS:
   Is necessary for digestive function.   T
   Usually has long preganglionic efferent nerve fibres.   T
   Uses acetylcholine as its major neurotransmitter.   T
   Operates through nicotinic and muscarinic ACh receptors.   T
4. PNS stimulation:
   Causes pupillary dilation.   F
       Causes pupillary constriction.
   Causes increased salivation.   T
   Increases heart rate and force of contraction.   F
       Decreases heart rate and force of contraction.
   Increases bronchial secretions.   T
   Promotes GIT motility.   T
   Inhibits bladder smooth muscle contraction.   F
       Stimulates bladder smooth muscle contraction.
   Blocks penile vasodilatation and erection.   F
       Stimulates penile vasodilatation and erection.
5. In the PNS, nicotinic ACh receptors occur in the ganglion.   T
6. In the PNS muscarinic ACh receptors occur in the ganglion.   T
7. In the PNS, muscarinic receptors occur on target tissues.   T
8. Ganglionic muscarinic receptors mediate postsynaptic recover after
   depolarisation of the neurone.   T
9. Postsynaptic ACh receptors regulate ACh release from nerves.   F
       Presynaptic ACh receptors regulate ACh release from the nerve.
10. M2 ACh muscarinic receptors occur in heart muscle.   T
11. Nicotinic agonists are used to treat Parkinsonism.   T

12. Pilocarpine, a muscarinic antagonist, is used to treat glaucoma.   F
    Pilocarpine, a muscarinic *agonist*, is used to treat glaucoma.
13. Atropine is a muscarinic antagonist.   T
14. Tropicamide is a short-acting antimuscarinic drug.   T
15. Anticholinergic drugs block the actions of atropine.   F
    Anticholinergic drugs block the actions of acetylcholine.
16. Anticholinergic drugs are used:
    As GIT antispasmodics.   T
    For motion sickness.   T
    To dilate the pupil for eye examinations.   T
    As premedication before operations.   T
    To treat polyuria.   F
    To treat urinary incontinence.
17. Anticholinesterase drugs block the action of acetylcholine.   F
    Anticholinesterase drugs block the action of *acetylcholinesterase*,
    thus prolonging cholinergic effects.
18. Anticholinesterase drugs:
    Cause slowing of the heart (bradycardia).   T
    Hypotension.   T
    Bronchoconstriction.   T
    Decreased peristalsis.   F
    Increased peristalsis.
    Fall in intraocular pressure.   T
19. Clinical uses of anticholinesterases include:
    Treatment of myasthenia gravis.   T
    Postoperative reversal of muscle relaxant action.   T
    Occasionally treatment of glaucoma.   T
    Treatment of Alzheimer's disease.   T

Chapter 9 Quiz answers

T = TRUE   F = FALSE

1. The SNS is not essential for life.   T
2. SNS efferent outflows are via the thoraco-lumbar cord segments.   T
3. The SNS:
    Is necessary for the flight or fight reflex.   T
    Usually has a short preganglionic efferent nerve fibre.   T
    Uses norepinephrine as its major neurotransmitter.   T
    Is highly selective in its physiological responses.   F
    Is relatively non-selective in its discharge responses.
4. SNS stimulation:
    Causes pupillary dilation through α_1-adrenoceptors.   T

Increases cardiac rate and force of contraction via β_1-adrenoceptors.   T

Causes bronchial constriction via β_2-adrenoceptors.   F

   Causes bronchial dilation via β_2-adrenoceptors.

Causes thermogenesis through lipolysis via β_3-adrenoceptors.   T

Constricts the bladder neck to inhibit urination.   T

Promotes non-pregnant uterine contractions.   F

   Promotes non-pregnant uterine relaxation via β_2-adrenoceptors.

Enables ejaculation via α_1-adrenoceptors.   T

5. In the SNS, nicotinic ACh receptors occur in the ganglion.   T

6. In the SNS, muscarinic ACh receptors occur in the ganglion.   T

7. In the SNS, muscarinic receptors occur on target tissues.   F

   In the SNS adrenergic receptors occur on target tissues.

8. Ganglionic muscarinic receptors mediate postsynaptic recovery after depolarisation of the neurone.   T

9. Presynaptic α_2-adrenoceptors inhibit NE release from nerves.   T

10. NE cause glycogenolysis in skeletal muscle via β_2-adrenoceptors.   T

11. NE action is terminated by Uptake 1 into presynaptic nerves.   T

12. Uptake 1 is enhanced by amphetamines.   F

   Uptake 1 is inhibited by amphetamines (and by tricyclics).

13. Oxymetazoline, used to relieve nasal congestion is an α_1-agonist.   T

14. NE and epinephrine are metabolised by MAO.   T

15. NE and epinephrine are also metabolised by COMT.   T

Chapter 10 Quiz answers

T = TRUE   F = FALSE

1. The motor endplate is postsynaptic on the muscle membrane.   T

2. The motor endplate is a target for neuromuscular blockers.   T

3. The main events at the NMJ resulting in ACh release are:

Arrival of the impulse at the motor nerve terminal, which   T

Triggers Ca^{2+} influx into the cytoplasm, which   T

Triggers fusion of vesicles with nerve cell membrane and   T

Release of epinephrine into the synaptic cleft.   F

   Release of *acetylcholine (ACh)* into the synaptic cleft.

4. The main NMJ postsynaptic events are:

Binding of ACh to ACh receptors on the motor endplate, which   T

Causes ion channel opening and Na^+ influx, which   T

Causes a transmembrane electrochemical gradient and   T

Generation of a local endplate potential, which   T

Spreads over the muscle fibre and triggers   T

A generalised release of intracellular Na^+ ions   F

   A release of intracellular Ca^{2+} from the SA.*

	Resulting in muscle contraction.	T
5.	The nicotinic NMJ ACh receptor has 2 ACh-binding α subunits.	T
6.	Non-depolarising NMJ blocking drugs:	
	Include aminosteroids and benzylisoquinolines.	T
	Are usually irreversibly bound to the ACh receptor.	F
	Are usually *reversibly* bound to the ACh receptor.	
	Are competitive antagonists of ACh at the ACh receptor.	T
	May bind also to presynaptic ACh receptors.	T
	Action duration depends mainly on systemic clearance.	T
	Have low potential for reactive hyperthermia.	T
	Action is reversed by increasing local ACh concentrations.	T
	Include pancuronium, rocuronium and vecuronium.	T
7.	Aminosteroids have high HIS[†] release potential.	F
	Have low *histamine* release potential.	
8.	They can cause sympathomimetic and vagolytic effects.	T
9.	These include tachycardia and hypertension.	T
10.	They have powerful analgesic or sedative action.	F
	They have little if any analgesic or sedative effects.	
11.	Benzylisoquinoline NMJ blocking drugs:	
	Include atracurium, cisatracurium, gallamine, mivacurium.	T
	Can cause histamine release with bradycardia and hypotension.	T
	Action is prolonged in patients with myasthenia gravis.	T
	Require dose titration with low plasma cholinesterase patients.	T
	Should be used with caution, if at all, in pregnant patients.	T
12.	Suxamethonium:	
	Is the only depolarising NMJ blocker used now.[‡]	T
	Consists of three molecules of ACh joined together.	F
	Consists of *two* molecules of ACh joined together.	
	On binding to the ACh receptor causes initial tremor before block.	T
	Is used when fast NMJ block is needed, e.g. emergency use.	T
	Is used when fast recovery from block is required.	T
	Should be administered after induction.[§]	T
	Should be avoided with penetrating eye injury.	T
	Is contraindicated with recent burn injuries.	T
	Can cause arrhythmias and cardiac arrest.	T
13.	Anticholinesterase drugs:	
	Enhance the breakdown of ACh by acetylcholinesterase.	F
	Anticholinesterases *block* the breakdown of ACh.	
	May be reversible or irreversible.	T
	Are used to treat myasthenia gravis by prolonging NMJ ACh action.	T
	Are used to treat Alzheimer's disease.	T
14.	Reversible anticholinesterases may be:	
	Short-acting, e.g. neostigmine.	F
	Neostigmine is *not* short-acting; **edrophonium** is the answer here.	
	Of medium duration, e.g. rivastigmine.	T

Used to diagnose and treat myasthenia gravis.	T
Used to treat open-angle glaucoma.	T
Used to re-activate the GIT after surgery.	T

---

* SA Sarcoplasmic reticulum.
† HIS: histamine.
‡ At the time of writing.
§ Tremors or fasciculation caused by suxamethonium before block can be painful.

Chapter 11 Quiz answers

T = TRUE   F = FALSE

1. Myasthenia gravis (MG) is a debilitating disease of smooth muscle.	F
Voluntary muscle.	
2. MG is an autoimmune disease that targets the NMJ.*	T
3. Important targets for antibody production include:	
The acetylcholine receptor at the NMJ.	T
Nerve-specific tyrosine kinase (MuSK).	F
Muscle-specific tyrosine kinase.	
4. Symptoms of myasthenia gravis include:	
Drooping eyelids (ptosis).	T
Double vision (diplopia).	T
Speech difficulties (dysarthria).	T
Difficulty swallowing (dysphagia).	T
Generalised muscle weakness.	T
Respiratory distress.	T
5. Antibodies block ACh binding to its receptor at the NMJ.	T
6. Diagnostic procedures include:	
Detection of circulating antibodies to the ACh receptor.	T
ECG.	F
Electromyography.	
Detection of circulating antibodies to MuSK.†	T
7. Treatment of myasthenia gravis employs:	
Anticholinesterases displace antibodies from ACh receptors.	F
Anticholinesterases increase ACh concentrations in the synapse.	
Immunosuppressants e.g. corticosteroids.	T
Plasmapheresis.	T
Thymectomy.	T
8. Juvenile myasthenia gravis may be diagnosed using edrophonium.	T
9. Juvenile MG has similar treatment strategies as for adults.	T
10. Lambert-Eaton myasthenic syndrome (LEMS) involves lack of ACh.	F

Involves autoimmune attack on presynaptic voltage-gated Ca^{2+} channels.

11. LEMS requires drugs that potentiate ACh release and action.   T

---

* NMJ: neuromuscular junction.
† MuSK: muscle-specific tyrosine kinase.

Chapter 12 Quiz answers

T = TRUE   F = FALSE

1. 5-HT occurs mainly in liver, CNS and gut.   F
     5-HT occurs mainly in *platelets*, CNS and gut.
2. 5-HT is synthesised from dietary tryptophan.   T
3. Synthesis is regulated by tyrosine hydroxylase.   F
     Tryptophan hydroxylase (tyrosine hydroxylase regulates
     norepinephrine synthesis).
4. 5-HT is a CNS neurotransmitter mediating (e.g.):   T
   Sleep-waking patterns.   T
   Brain reward pathways.   T
   Vomiting reflex.   T
   Mood.   T
   Migraine.   T
   Body temperature regulation.   T
5. 5-HT action is terminated by postsynaptic uptake.   F
     Presynaptic uptake by SERTs.*
6. SERTs are targets for drugs that enhance 5-HT action at the synapse.   T
7. 5-HT is metabolised to 5-hydroxyindole acetic acid, excreted in the   T
   urine.
8. 5-HT autoreceptors on postsynaptic cells promote further synthesis of   F
   5-HT.
     5-HT autoreceptors on *presynaptic nerve endings inhibit* 5-HT
     neurotransmitter activity.
9. 5-HT is a relatively unimportant neurotransmitter and modulator in the   F
   GIT.
     5-HT is a *major* neuromodulator and neurotransmitter in the GIT.

---

* Serotonin-selective re-uptake transporters.

Chapter 13 Quiz answers

T = TRUE   F = FALSE

1. *Eiconasoids* is a collective term for 20-carbon fatty acids.   T
2. Eiconasoids include prostanoids, leukotrienes and thromboxane.   T
3. Prostaglandins:
   Are derived from arachidonic acid.   T
   Mediate pain and inflammation.   T
   Are involved in the process of implantation in the uterus.   T
   Actions are blocked by paracetamol.   F
     Actions are blocked by aspirin.
4. Leukotrienes:
   Are important mediators of bronchial constriction.   T
   Are synthesised through the action of cyclooxegenase enzymes.   F
     Lipoxygenase enzymes.
   Mediate increased capillary permeability.   T
   Mediate fast hypersensitivity responses.   T
   Inhibit chemotaxis.   F
     Promote chemotaxis.
5. LTC4, LTD4 and LTE4 are cystinyl leukotrienes.   T
6. Prostaglandin PGD_2 mediates bronchoconstriction, for example.   T
7. PGE_2 enhances gastric mucosa breakdown.   F
     PGE_2 *protects* gastric mucosa from breakdown.
8. $PGF_2\alpha$ mediates pain and inflammation.   T
9. Aspirin blocks prostaglandin production.   T
10. Prostacyclin (PGI_2) inhibits platelet aggregation.   T
11. Prostacyclin is used to treat pulmonary hypertension.   T
12. Leukotriene-modifying drugs are used to treat asthma.   T

Chapter 14 Quiz answers

T = TRUE   F = FALSE

1. A chimaeric drug is constructed from more than one species.   T
2. Monoclonal antibodies are derived from a single B cell clone.   T
3. Erythropoietin stimulates white cell production.   F
     It stimulates *red* cell production.
4. Polypeptides and proteins are formed via peptide bonds.   T
5. TNF-α is a target for biological drugs.   T
6. Abciximab is used to treat rheumatoid arthritis.   F

In blood vessel repair as it blocks platelet aggregation.

7.	Erythropoietin is used to treat anaemia.	T
8.	Etanercept is used to treat rheumatoid arthritis.	T
9.	Synthetic growth hormone is used preferentially.*	T
10.	Interferons are produced by cells under bacterial attack.	F
	They are produced by cells under *viral* attack.	
11.	Trastuzumab is used to treat metastatic breast cancer.	T
12.	Vasopressin is used to treat diabetes mellitus.	F
	Diabetes *insipidus*.	
13.	Peptides and proteins as drugs may present problems involving:	
	Purification.	T
	Compromising patient immunity to infection.	T
	Immunogenic potential of the drug.	T
	Adverse effects.	T
	Administration of the drug.	T
	Production and storage.	T
14.	The quaternary structure of a protein is the amino acid sequence.	F
	It is the structure determined by the arrangement of protein subunits.	

* To avoid dangers of contamination with, for example, HIV.

Chapter 16 Quiz answers

T = TRUE   F = FALSE

1.	Mannitol is useful in surgery to maintain renal function.	T
2.	Mannitol increases the osmolality of urine.	T
3.	Carbonic anhydrase inhibitors decrease urinary bicarbonate.	F
	They increase urinary bicarbonate.	
4.	Acetazolamide may be used to treat aspirin poisoning.	T
5.	Thiazides act at the glomerulus to enhance chloride excretion.	F
	Thiazides block Cl^- reabsorption in the distal tubule.	
6.	Thiazide-like drugs include chlortalidone.	T
7.	Thiazides have moderate diuretic potency.	T
8.	Thiazides may be used to manage mild to moderate heart failure.	T
9.	Adverse effects of thiazides include hypoglycaemia.	F
	Adverse effects include *hyperglycaemia.*	
10.	Thiazides are contraindicated in Addison's disease.	T
11.	Loop diuretics:	
	Block Cl^- reabsorption in the glomerulus.	F
	In the thick part of the ascending Loop of Henle.	
	Result in small volumes of hypertonic urine presented to the tubules.	F
	Result in *large* volumes of *hypotonic* urine.	

12. Loop diuretics include bumetanide and furosemide.   T
13. Loop diuretics are used for hypertension.   T
14. Loop diuretics can cause bone marrow suppression.   T
15. Spirinolactone blocks aldosterone action in the adrenal gland.   F
     In the distal tubule by blocking the aldosterone receptor.
16. Clinical uses of spirinolactone include oedema of liver cirrhosis.   T
17. Thiazide diuretics are contraindicated in patients with gout.   T

Chapter 17 Quiz answers

T = TRUE   F = FALSE

1. Afterload is arterial resistance against which the heart has to pump.   T
2. Preload is venous back pressure.   T
3. Diseased heart responds to stretch with increased contractility.   F
     The diseased heart is *unable* to respond to stretch with increased contraction.
4. The diseased heart becomes enlarged.   T
5. Heart failure may be caused by hypothyroidism.   F
     It may be caused by thyrotoxicosis.
6. Patients with heart failure cannot exercise effectively.   T
7. Oedema and kidney failure are associated with heart failure.   T
8. Treatment aims to restore cardiac ability to obey Starling's Law.   T
9. Treatment aims to increase the heart's workload.   F
     Treatment aims to *decrease* the heart's workload.
10. Treatment aims to decrease preload and oedema.   T
11. ACE inhibitors block the breakdown of angiotensin-II.   F
     ACE inhibitors block the *formation* of angiotensin-II.
12. β-blockers help by increasing sympathetic tone to the heart.   F
     β-blockers help by *decreasing* sympathetic tone.
13. Diuretics help by reducing oedema water and salt.   T
14. Vasodilators, for example, nitroprusside help by reducing preload.   T
15. Digoxin restores the heart's ability to obey Starling's Law.   T
16. ACE inhibitors are contraindicated with renovascular disease.   T
17. Caution! ACE inhibitors potentiate diuretics.   T
18. Thiazide diuretics are contraindicated in patients with gout.   T
19. Loop diuretics block $Na^+/K^+/Cl^-$ reabsorption in the collecting ducts.   F
     In the ascending limb of the Loop of Henle.
20. β-blockers are contraindicated in asthmatic patients.   T
21. β- blockers may reduce mortality in patients with left-ventricular systolic dysfunction.   T

Chapter 18 Quiz answers

T = TRUE   F = FALSE

1. Heart block is failure of impulse conduction in cardiac tissue.   T
2. Cardiopulmonary resuscitation is emergency chest compression and
   mouth-to-mouth ventilation.   T
3. Thrombolysis is dissolving of a blood clot.   T
4. Risk factors for myocardial infarction include:
   Hypertension.   T
   Anorexia.   F
      Obesity.
5. Ventricular tachycardia (VT is an early complication of a heart attack.   T
6. VT can develop into ventricular fibrillation unless treated.   T
7. Symptoms of myocardial infarction include:
   Intense pain into arms and throat.   T
   Breathlessness.   T
   Anxiety and sweating.   T
   Perhaps no symptoms.   T
8. Diagnosis includes ECG and medical history.   T
9. Pharmacological interventions include:
   Oxygen.   T
   Dispersible aspirin.   T
   Streptokinase.   T
   IV diamorphine (heroin) or morphine.   T
   Heparin.   T
   Amiodarone.   T
   Fluid resuscitation.   T
10. Percutaneous coronary intervention is a procedure to widen coronary
    arteries.   T
11. Platelet aggregation inhibitors include:
    Clopidogrel.   T
    GPIIb/IIIa receptor antagonists.   T
12. Follow-up treatment for myocardial infarction includes:
    Regular low-dose aspirin.   T
    A statin.   T
    ACE inhibitors.   T
    β-blockers.   T

Chapter 19 Quiz answers

T = TRUE   F = FALSE

1. Normal cardiac rhythm is:
    Controlled by the sino-atrial node and by autonomic inputs to the SA
    node.   T
    Achieved through spread of electrical impulses through conducting
    tissues to atrial and ventricular muscles.   T
2. Arrhythmias:
    Are deviations from normal sinus rhythm.   T
    May be normal, temporary physiological responses.   T
    Always occur continuously.   F
        They may be continuous or intermittent.
    Produce symptoms of chest pain and 'palpitations'.   T
    May in some cases be potentially life-threatening.   T
3. Automaticity is caused by impulses from the S-A node.   F
        Local initiation of an ectopic focus anywhere in heart muscle.
4. The aims of drug treatment are:
    To slow the heart and restore normal rhythm.   T
    To correct abnormal pacemaker activity.   T
5. Antidysrythmic drugs are classified according to:
    Their chemical structure.   F
    Their site of action in the heart, for example supraventricular.   T
    Their mechanism of action.   T
6. Disopyramide and procainamide block fast Na^+ channels, which
    prolongs the duration of the action potential.   T
7. They are usually reserved for supraventricular tachycardia.   T
8. Lidocaine and mexiletine shorten action potential duration.   T
9. They are used for life-threatening ventricular arrhythmias.   T
10. Flecainide and propafenone lower rate of depolarisation of the AP.*   T
11. Lidocaine is used for emergencies, for example a heart attack.   T
12. Lidocaine doses should be reduced after heart surgery or with CHF.   T
13. Flecainide is used for:
    Treatment and prevention of paroxysmal atrial tachycardia.   T
    Prevention of suspected life-threatening ventricular tachycardia.   T
    Arrhythmias associated with Wolff-Parkinson-White syndrome.   T
14. Flecainide is contraindicated in patients with a history of MI.   T
15. Propranolol is a Class I antidysrhythmic drug.   F
        β-blockers are *Class II*.
16. β-blockers are contradicted in patients with asthma.   T
17. Amiodarone is a Class III antidysrhythmic drug.   T
18. Amiodarone may cause thyroid dysfunction.   T
19. Amiodarone is used to resuscitate during ventricular fibrillation.   T

20. Verapamil is used to treat supraventricular tachycardias.   T
21. Verapamil is contraindicated in patients with a history of heart failure.   T
22. Verapamil is a K^+ channel blocker.   F
     Ca^{2+} L-type ion channel blocker.
23. Digoxin has a very narrow margin of safety.   T
24. Digoxin slows the heart by suppressing vagal drive to it.   F
     Enhancing vagal drive to the heart.
25. Low plasma K^+ increases digoxin toxicity.   T
26. Digoxin blood levels should be monitored during treatment.   T
27. Adenosine is a pyrimidine nucleotide.   F
     Adenosine is a purine nucleoside.
28. Adenosine is the treatment of choice for terminating paroxysmal
     supraventricular tachycardia.   T

---

* AP: action potential.

Chapter 20 Quiz answers

T = TRUE   F = FALSE

1. Angina pectoris is chest pain caused by inadequate O_2 supply to heart
    muscle.   T
2. Symptoms are crushing pain and suffocating chest sensations.   T
3. Risk factors for angina pectoris include:
    Diabetes.   T
    Family history of angina.   T
    Hypercholesterolaemia.   T
    A sedentary lifestyle.   T
    Hypotension.   F
       Hypertension.
4. Triggers for angina pectoris include:
    Sudden, sustained physical exertion.   T
    Emotional stress.   T
    Dreams.   T
    After a meal.   T
5. Unstable angina may herald an imminent heart attack.   T
6. Diagnostic procedures for angina include:
    ECG.   T
       Fasting glucose.   F
    Monitoring heart rate and rhythm during exercise.   T
    Thallium scintigram.   T
    Coronary angiogram.   T

7. Aims of treatment include:
    Prevent and stop the pain. T
    Reduce rate of atheroma deposition. T
    Reduce the risk of myocardial infarction. T
    Introduce lifestyle changes. T
    More strenuous exercise. F
        Absolutely NOT; gentle exercise recommended.
8. Drug treatments include:
    Symptomatic relief with glyceryl trinitrate. T
    Use of longer-acting nitrates, for example isosorbide dinitrate. T
    Dyhydropyridine-based Ca^{2+}-channel blockers. T
    Statins to slow atheroma formation in coronary arteries. T
9. Unstable angina:
    When diagnosed requires immediate admission as an emergency. T
    Requires ECG monitoring. T
    May require heparin infusion and aspirin. T
    May require IIb/IIIa inhibitors, for example tirofiban or eptifibatide. T
    May require cardiac catheterisation. T

Chapter 21 Quiz answers

T = TRUE   F = FALSE

1. Platelets are used to widen arteries. F
        Platelets are bodies in blood involved in haemostasis.
2. Infarction is death of tissue through interrupted blood supply. T
3. Thrombocytopaenia is an excess of platelets. F
        A *deficiency* of platelets in blood.
4. Platelets are activated by:
    Epinephrine. T
    Adhesion to collagen. T
    Contact with fibrinogen. T
    Contact with ADP. T
    Contact with thrombin. T
    Contact with glass. T
5. When activated inhibit thromboxane (TxA_2) synthesis. F
        Activated platelets increase TXA_2 production.
6. Platelets are biosynthesised mainly in bone marrow. T
7. Aspirin in low doses inhibits platelet activation by blocking TxA_2 T
    synthesis.
8. Aspirin is non-allergic. F
        Aspirin *is* potentially allergic as a hapten (*see* Mini glossary).

9. Clopidogrel inhibits platelet aggregation by enhancing ADP receptor activation.   F
   Clopidogrel *inhibits* ADP binding to its platelet ADP receptor.
10. Abciximab inhibits platelet activation by blocking the GPIIb/IIIA receptor.   T
11. Abciximab should not be used if there is a pre-existing bleeding risk.   T
12. Eptifibatide is an anticoagulant factor derived from the venom of a snake.   T
13. Tirofiban is a non-peptide antiplatelet drug given by IV infusion.   T

Chapter 22 Quiz answers

T = TRUE   F = FALSE

1. Coagulation is the conversion of liquid to solid blood.   T
2. Is initiated by tissue damage or blood contact with, for example, glass.   T
3. Coagulation is a target for drugs that treat, for example:
   Atrial fibrillation.   T
   Deep venous thrombosis.   T
   Pulmonary embolism.   T
   Stable angina.   F
   Unstable angina.
4. Heparin:
   Is chemically a glycosaminoglycan.   T
   Is produced by basophils and mast cells.   T
   Inactivates thrombin and factor Xa.   T
   Potentiates antithrombin (AT-III) activity 1000-fold.   T
   Is inactivated by heparinase enzymes.   T
   Has a long half-life.   F
   Has a *short* half-life (± 1 hour)
   Carries a serious risk of thrombocytopaenia.   T
   Carries a risk of osteoporosis with long-term use.   T
5. Heparin is used for:
   Prophylaxis in orthopaedic surgery.   T
   Thrombocytopaenia.   F
   Certainly NOT; Heparin may cause thrombocytopaenia.
   Pulmonary embolism.   T
   Management of myocardial infarction.   T
   Management of acute peripheral arterial occlusion.   T
   Procedures that require a quickly reversible anticoagulant.   T
   Rapid treatment of deep venous thrombosis.   T

6. LMWH* need more frequent dosage than unfractionated heparin.   F
   Require less frequent dosage.
7. LMWH are prepared by fractionating native heparin.   T
8. LMWH need be given once daily only by SC injection.   T
9. LMWH usually carry a greater bleeding risk than does heparin.   F
   LMWH may carry a smaller bleeding risk.
10. LMWH:
   Include bemiparin, dalteparin, enoxaparin, reviparin, tinzaparin.   T
   Carry a smaller risk of thrombocytopaenia than does heparin.   T
   Carry a lesser risk of osteoporosis with long-term use.   T
   Can be used with out-patients.   T
11. LMWH have generally similar precautions for use as heparin.   T
12. Hirudins are anticoagulants derived from the skin of a frog.   F
   Hirudins are derived from the salivary glands of the leech.
13. Lepirudin is recombinant hirudin.   T
14. Hirudins bind to and inactivate the active form of thrombin.   T
15. Hirudins are used for patients who cannot take heparin.   T
16. Hirudins also lyse the blot clot.   T
17. Hirudins are contraindicated in pregnancy.   T
18. Hirudins require caution in patients with liver or kidney problems.   T
19. Danaparoid sodium is a heparinoid derived from heparin.   T
20. Fondaparinux is an anticoagulant that inactivates activated
   factor X.   T
21. Protamine sulphate is an antidote for heparin.   T

---

* LMH: low molecular weight heparins.

Chapter 23 Quiz answers

T = TRUE   F = FALSE

1. Oral anticoagulants are taken by mouth.   T
2. Have a delayed onset of action.   T
3. Warfarin:
   Blocks active vitamin K biosynthesis.   T
   Can be taken by the patient at home.   T
   Is associated with extensive drug interactions.   T
   Is a fat-soluble vitamin   F
   Vitamin K is a fat-soluble vitamin.
4. Warfarin action is potentiated by:
   Inhibitors of liver microsomal enzymes.   T
   Some antibiotics, e.g. ciprofloxaxin.   T
   Vitamin K.   F

Warfarin inhibits vitamin K action		
Antidepressants, e.g. imipramine.		T
H2-receptor blockers, e.g. cimetidine.		T
Cephalosporins, which inhibit vitamin K reduction.		T
Inhibitors of platelet function, e.g. aspirin.		T
5.	Adverse effects of warfarin include:	
	Haemorrhage.	T
	Fall in haematocrit.	T
	Liver disorders.	T
	Pancreatitis.	T
	Osteoporosis with prolonged use.	T
	Thrombocytopaenia.	T
	Hypersensitivity reactions.	T
6.	Contraindications with warfarin include:	
	Alcoholism.	T
	Severe hypertension.	T
	First and third trimesters of pregnancy.	T
	Recent CNS surgery.	T
	Bacterial endocarditis.	T
	Bleeding disorders, e.g. peptic ulcer.	T
7.	Precautions with warfarin include:	
	Breast-feeding.	T
	Pregnancy.	T
	Impaired pituitary function.	F
	Impaired *liver and kidney* function.	

Chapter 24 Quiz answers

T = TRUE   F = FALSE

1.	Fibrinolysis is digestion of fibrin.	T
2.	Plasmin is a proteolytic enzyme formed from plasminogen.	T
3.	Plasmin is produced from kallikrein.	F
	Plasmin is produced from plasminogen.	
4.	Plasmin cuts specifically arginine and lysine C-terminal junctions.	T
5.	Antifibrinolytic drugs inhibit fibrinolysis.	T
6.	Antifibrinolytic drugs are used to promote bleeding.	F
	Antifibrinolytic drugs are used to *prevent* bleeding.	
7.	Antifibrinolytics help to control bleeding during surgery.	T
8.	Aprotinin is a serine protease inhibitor.	T
9.	Aprotinin is administered mainly by IV infusion or injection.	T
10.	Tranexamic acid is extracted from platelets.	F
	Tranexamic acid is a synthetic drug.	

11. Tranexamic acid inhibits conversion of plasminogen to plasmin.   T
12. Tranexamic acid cannot be administered orally.   F
    Tranexamic acid is administered orally or by IV injection.
13. Fibrinolytic drugs promote break-down of the fibrin clot.   T
14. Fibrinolytic drugs activate plasminogen to form plasmin.   T
15. Streptokinase is a first generation fibrinolytic drug.   T
16. Streptokinase is currently indicated mainly for life-threatening cases.   T
17. Streptokinase converts plasmin to plasminogen.   F
    Streptokinase converts plasminogen to plasmin.
18. Streptokinase is an enzyme derived from streptococcus.   T
19. Streptokinase is used, for example, in acute myocardial infarction.   T
20. Alteplase is also known as rt-PA.   T
21. Alteplase binds to fibrin.   T
22. The alteplase-fibrin complex converts plasminogen to plasmin.   T
23. 3rd generation fibrinolytics are more specific for clot-bound fibrin.   T

Chapter 25 Quiz answers

T = TRUE   F = FALSE

1. Systolic pressure is due to heart contraction.   T
2. Diastolic pressure is due to the arterial resistance to blood flow.   T
3. Blood pressure is expressed in mmHg (mercury).   T
4. Blood pressure is normally controlled by:
   Rate and force of cardiac contraction.   T
   Activity of the RAAS* system.   T
   Resistance offered by the peripheral blood vessels.   T
   The baroreceptor reflex.   T
   Diet.   F
      Poor diet can contribute to risk factors for hypertension.
5. Abnormally high diastolic pressure may reflect hypertension.   T
6. Persistently raised BP (e.g. 140/90 mmHg) reflects hypertension.   T
7. Possible consequences of persistent hypertension include:
   Hypertensive cardiomyopathy.   T
   Increased risk of myocardial infarction.   T
   Hypertensive retinopathy.   T
   Hypertensive nephropathy.   T
   Syncope (fainting).   F
      Syncope is more usually associated with hypotension.
8. Diagnostic tools for hypertension include:
   Measurement of blood pressure.   T
   Blood tests for abnormally high catecholamines.[†]   T

Measurement of plasma K^+, Na^+ and creatinine.[‡]   T

Measurement of blood glucose (test for diabetes).   T

---

* Renin-angiotensin-aldosterone system.

† To distinguish essential from secondary hypertension.

‡ Check for kidney damage.

Chapter 26 Quiz answers

T = TRUE   F = FALSE

1. Treat with antihypertensives if BP 140/90 + no organ damage + no cardiovascular complications.   F
     Lifestyle + dietary counselling; no drugs + monthly check-ups.
2. Lifestyle counselling advice involves:
   Weight reduction.   T
   Exercise if possible.   T
   Reduce salt, alcohol and fatty food intake.   T
   Stop smoking.   T
3. The aims of drug treatment are:
   In most cases to keep blood pressure below 140/90 mmHg.   T
   For diabetics or patients with renal disease, below 120/80.   T
4. Drugs used include:
   Aspirin.   F
     Aspirin lowers temperature, not blood pressure.
   Thiazide diuretics.   T
   Heparin.   F
     Heparin prolongs clotting time.
   ACE inhibitors.   T
   Angiotensin-II receptor antagonists.   T
   Calcium channel blockers.   T
   Centrally acting drugs, e.g. clonidine.   T
   Direct vasodilators.   T
   β-adrenoceptor agonists.   F
     β-adrenoceptor *antagonists.*
5. For young white patients, ACE inhibitors are initial choices.   T
6. ACE inhibitors may not be effective in Black patients initially.   T
7. β-blockers are favoured initially for uncomplicated hypertension.   F
     β-blockers are *not* favoured as initial treatment for uncomplicated hypertension (at time of writing).
8. Diltiazem and verapamil are usually suitable for angina patients.   T
9. α-blockers are used only in very resistant cases of hypertension.   T

10. ARBs are useless in patients intolerant to ACE inhibitors.   F
    ARBS are *useful* for patients intolerant to ACE inhibitors.
11. Thiazide diuretics inhibit $Na^+/-Cl^-$ reabsorption in distal tubules.   T
12. Thiazides are often first line of treatment in newly diagnosed
    hypertension.   T
13. Thiazides may cause hyperglycaemia and Hyperuricaemia.   T
14. Thiazides should not be used in patient's with Addison's disease.   T
15. β-blockers are contraindicated in:
    Asthmatic patients.   T
    Uncontrolled heart failure.   T
    Hypotension.   T
    Prinzmetal's angina.   T
16. Direct vasodilators stimulate ACh receptors on smooth muscle.   F
    Direct vasodilators act directly on smooth muscle to relax it,
    for example hydralazine inhibits free radical formation; sodium
    nitroprusside is a source of nitric oxide.
17. Adverse effects with hydralazine include:
    Arrhythmias.   T
    Hypotension.   T
    Thrombocytopaenia.   T
    Leucopaenia.   T
    Hair loss.   F
    Hirsutism has been reported.
18. Sodium nitroprusside can cause precipitous hypotension.   T
19. ACE inhibitors are:
    A good first line treatment with young Caucasians.   T
    Favoured for patients with IDDM and nephropathies.   T
    Prophylactic against stroke after myocardial infarction.   T
    Available only in injectable form.   F
    Available as oral tablets.
    Contraindicated in patients with renovascular disease.   T
20. Angiotensin-II receptor blockers include:
    Candesartan.   T
    Eprosartan.   T
    Captopril.   F
    Captopril is an ACE inhibitor.
21. Calcium channel blockers include:
    Amlopidine.   T
    Diltiazem.   T
    Nifedipine.   T
    Verapamil.   T
    Nicorandil.   F
    Nicorandil is an anti-angina drug.
22. Ca^{2+}-channel blockers block L-type voltage-gated Ca^{2+} channels.   T
23. Ca^{2+}-channel blockers are used as prophylaxis against angina.   T

24. Ca^{2+}-channel blockers are used to treat hypertension, e.g. diltiazem. T
25. Ca^{2+}-channel blockers may cause bradycardia and syncope. T

Chapter 27 Quiz answers

T = TRUE   F = FALSE

1. Inflammation is the tissue response to damaging stimuli. T
2. Inflammation has two phases, acute and chronic. T
3. The acute phase involves angiogenesis and tissue destruction. F
   The chronic phase involves angiogenesis and tissue destruction.
4. Important chemical mediators of inflammation include:
   Histamine. T
   5-HT. T
   Norepinephrine. F
   Prostaglandins. T
   Leukotrienes. T
   TNF-α. T
5. Type I hypersensitivity:
   Is antibody-mediated. F
   Is an allergic response to allergens, for example eggs and pollen.
   Chemical mediators include histamine and 5-HT. T
   Reactions present with, for example, oedema, hay fever, and itch. T
   Can result in anaphylactic shock. T
   Reactions may be treated with antihistamines. T
6. Type 2 hypersensitivity:
   Is antibody-mediated. T
   Causes thyroid problems. T
7. Type 3 hypersensitivity:
   Involves deposition in tissue of immune complexes. T
   Mediates the Arthus reaction. T
   Mediates reactions to poison ivy. F
   Poison ivy involves a Type 4 hypersensitivity response.
   Mediates rheumatoid arthritis. T

Chapter 28 Quiz answers

T = TRUE   F = FALSE

1. Aspirin is anti-inflammatory by stimulating biosynthesis of
   prostaglandins. F

Aspirin *inhibits* biosynthesis of the prostaglandins.

2. NSAIDs are used to treat symptomatic pain and inflammation.   T
3. Aspirin is poorly absorbed rectally in suppository form.   F
   Aspirin is *well* absorbed rectally.
4. NSAIDs are used to treat arthritic pain.   T
5. Aspirin is contraindicated for patients at risk of heart diseases.   F
   Aspirin at low dose (75 mg) is prophylactic against myocardial
   infarction.
6. Aspirin is relatively well absorbed from the stomach.   T
7. Aspirin is well absorbed from the small gut despite the alkaline Ph.   T
8. Aspirin is largely reabsorbed from alkaline urine.   F
   Aspirin is excreted faster in alkaline urine as more of it is in charged
   form.
9. At therapeutic doses aspirin causes GIT bleeding.   T
10. Acute renal failure is an adverse effect of aspirin.   T
11. There is risk of myocardial infarction with NSAIDs.   T
12. NSAIDs are best avoided during the third trimester of pregnancy.   T

Chapter 29 Quiz answers

T = TRUE   F = FALSE

1. Cortisol is the most potent physiological glucocorticoid.   T
2. Synthetic glucocorticoids vary in potency.   T
3. Anti-inflammatory actions of glucocorticoids include:
   Inhibition of prostaglandin synthesis.   T
   Activating lipocortin.   T
   Inhibiting release of inflammatory cytokines.   T
   Promoting phagocytosis.   F
      Glucocorticoids *inhibit* phagocytosis.
4. Normal control of cortisol release involves:
   Hypothalamic CRH.   T
   Which promotes pituitary ACTH release.   T
   Which promotes adrenal cortisol release.   T
   Inhibition of CRH and ACTH release by cortisol.   T
   Which promotes further cortisol release.   F
      This *inhibits* further cortisol release.
5. Anti-inflammatory actions of glucocorticoids involve:
   Inhibition of eiconasoid biosynthesis.   T
   Inactivation of lipocortin activity.   F
      Activation of lipocortin activity.
   Inhibition of chemotaxis.   T
   Inhibition of phagocytosis.   T

	Inhibition of inflammatory cytokine release.	T
6.	Cortisol mechanism involves *de novo* protein synthesis.	T
7.	Beclomethasone is available in inhalation form.	T
8.	Glucocorticoids can be administered into an inflamed joint.	T
9.	Glucocorticoids are not taken orally.	F
	Glucocorticoids can be taken orally.	
10.	Patients on high dose glucocorticoids have special requirements, for example:	
	Gradual withdrawal from the drug.	T
	Surgical team prior knowledge that they are on glucocorticoids.	T
	Possibly higher drug doses when ill.	T
	Regular monitoring for adverse reactions.	T
11.	Adverse reactions include:	
	Hypertrophy of the adrenal cortex.	F
	Atrophy of the adrenal cortex.	
	Oedema and redistribution of body fat.	T
	Osteoporosis and bone thinning.	T
	Suppression of the immune system.	T
	Depression.	F
	More usually euphoria.	
	Suppression of a hypothalamic CRH-ACTH axis.	T

Chapter 30 Quiz answers

T = TRUE   F = FALSE

1.	DMARDs are disease-modifying antirheumatic drugs.	T
2.	Antimalarial drugs are used to treat SLE.	T
3.	Important diseases targeted by DMARDs include:	
	Rheumatoid arthritis.	T
	Crohn's disease.	T
	Sjögren's syndrome.	T
	Influenza.	F
	Influenza is not a rheumatic condition.	
4.	DMARDs currently comprise:	
	Antimalarial drugs.	T
	Drugs which interfere with nucleic acid synthesis.	T
	Drugs which inhibit or block inflammatory cytokines.	T
	Drugs which primarily block second messengers.	F
5.	Gold and penicillamine have been used as DMARDs.	T
6.	Currently used inhibitors of nucleic acid synthesis include:	
	Azathioprine.	T
	Leflunomide.	T

Methotrexate.	T
Aspirin.	F
Aspirin blocks prostaglandin synthesis.	

7. Currently used antimalarial drugs include:

Quinidine.	F
Quinidine is a an anti-arrhythmic drug.*	
Chloroquine.	T
Hydroxychloroquine.	T
Mepacrine.	T

8. Patients on antimalarials need regular checks for visual acuity. — T
9. Nucleic acid inhibitors can depress bone marrow function. — T
10. Patients on methotrexate should avoid folic acid. — F
    Patients on methotrexate should be given folic acid as a supplement.
11. Cytokine inhibitors are genetically engineered proteins. — T
12. Anakinra is designed to inactivate TNF-α. — F
    Anakinra inactivates IL-1.
13. Infliximab is administered by continuous IV infusion. — T
14. Adalimumab is designed to block TNF-α. — T
15. Patients on cytokine inhibitors may develop opportunistic fungal or
    bacterial infections. — T

---

* Quinidine is now listed as discontinued in the BNF.

Chapter 31 Quiz answers

T = TRUE   F = FALSE

1. Gout is caused by an abnormally slow rate of urate excretion. — T
2. Gout is an inflammatory reaction to urate deposition. — T
3. Gout often occurs in the knuckles when it is called *podagra*. — F
   The big toe.
4. Gout is characterised by symptoms including:

Burning pain at sites of urate deposition.	T
Discharging skin eruptions.	T
Lowered blood viscosity.	F
Raised blood viscosity.	
Raised ESR and CRP.	T
Tophi.	T

5. Treatments for gout include:

Antibiotics.	F
Anti-inflammatory drugs.	T
Colchicine.	T

	Allopurinol.	T
	Probenecid.	T
6.	Adverse effects of probenecid include:	
	Hair loss.	F
	Alopecia.	
	Anaemia.	T
	GIT upsets.	T
	Nephrotic syndrome.	T
	Urticaria.	T
	Pruritis.	T
7.	Scleroderma is caused by a bacterial infection.	F
	Scleroderma is an autoimmune disease.	
8.	Scleroderma may be:	
	Localised cutaneous.	T
	Diffuse cutaneous.	T
	Diffuse systemic.	T
9.	Raynaud's phenomenon is extreme cold in fingers.	T
10.	Raynaud's phenomenon may be caused by:	
	Vasodilation of finger arterioles.	F
	Vasoconstriction of arterioles.	
	Vinyl chloride.	T
	Occupational damage to hands.	T
	Underlying presence of scleroderma.	T
11.	Treatment of Raynaud's phenomenon includes:	
	Vasoconstrictors.	F
	Vasodilators, for example calcium channel antagonists.	
	Warm gloves.	T
	Changing from jobs which aggravate the problem.	T
12.	Treatment of cutaneous scleroderma includes:	
	Creams and ointments to soften and moisturise skin.	T
	Dietary supplements of vitamin D.	T
	Treatment of any oesophageal symptoms.	T
13.	Treatment of diffuse advanced scleroderma includes:	
	Immunosuppressants, e.g. cyclophosphamide.	T
	Anti-thymocyte globulin.	T
	Proton pump inhibitors, e.g. ranitidine.	F
	Should be, for example, omeprazole; ranitidine is an H2 antagonist.	
14.	Patients with advanced scleroderma may need antiarrhythmic drugs.	T

Chapter 32 Quiz answers

T = TRUE   F = FALSE

1. Paracetamol is prescribed for pain and fever.   T
2. Paracetamol is similar in structure to aspirin.   T
3. Paracetamol preparations include:
    Oral tablets 500 mg.   T
    Suppositories.   T
    Oral paediatric solution.   T
    Topical cream.   F
        Paracetamol is *not* applied topically (to this author's knowledge).
    Solutions for IV infusion.   T
4. Paracetamol is highly effective as an anti-inflammatory.   F
        Paracetamol is *not* anti-inflammatory.
5. Paracetamol may be prescribed for:
    Headache.   T
    Rheumatic flare-ups.   F
        Paracetamol is *not* anti-inflammatory.
    Mild pyrexia.   T
    Migraine.   T
    Post-immunisation pyrexia.   T
    Brief febrile convulsions.   T
6. Adverse effects of paracetamol include skin rashes.   T
7. Paracetamol is well absorbed orally.   T
8. Paracetamol is excreted unmetabolised.   F
        Paracetamol is metabolised in the liver and excreted as harmless
        sulphates or glucuronides in the urine.
9. Is initially metabolised to a toxic intermediate.   T
10. Which is rendered harmless by addition of liver glutathione.   T
11. Paracetamol is toxic in overdose due to exhaustion of glutathione.   T
12. Liver enzyme-inducing drugs enhance paracetamol toxicity.   T
13. Children are less resistant to paracetamol toxicity.   F
        Children are more resistant.
14. Poisoning is asymptomatic for the first 24 hours.   T
15. Symptoms of paracetamol poisoning may include:
    Nausea and vomiting within 24 hours.   T
    Symptoms of liver damage after 24 hours.   T
    These symptoms include:
        − jaundice.   T
        − liver cell enzymes present in the circulation.   T
        − abdominal pain.   T
        − hyperglycaemia.   F

         − hypoglycaemia.
         − oliguria and kidney failure.   T
16. Treatment includes:
    Oral activated charcoal.   T
    Acetylcysteine.   T

Chapter 33 Quiz answers

T = TRUE   F = FALSE

1.	Pain is perceived at the site of tissue injury.	F
	Pain is perceived by the brain.	
2.	Interruption of nervous afferent pathways can abolish pain perception.	T
3.	Morphine blocks pain at the site of injury.	F
	Morphine blocks the brain's ability to appreciate pain.	
4.	Actions of morphine include:	
	CNS depression.	T
	Depression of pain awareness.	T
	Depression of respiration.	T
	Suppression of the cough reflex.	T
	Hypnotic.	T
	Euphoria.	T
	Depression of the vomiting centre.	F
	Stimulation of the vomiting centre.	
5.	Heroin is diethyl morphine.	F
	Heroin is *diacetyl* morphine.	
6.	A partial agonist may under some conditions become an antagonist.	T
7.	Codeine is used in cough mixtures.	T
8.	Codeine causes diarrhoea.	F
	Codeine constipates.	
9.	Heroin does not cross the blood−brain barrier.	F
	Heroin quickly crosses the blood−brain barrier.	
10.	Tolerance is when more drug is needed to obtain the same response.	T
11.	Psychological dependence is exhibited as drug-seeking behaviour.	T
12.	Physical dependence manifests itself through withdrawal symptoms.	T
13.	Naltrexone is used to wean addicts off morphine or heroin.	T

Chapter 34 Quiz answers

T = TRUE   F = FALSE

1. Local anaesthetics produce a local anaesthesia.   T
2. Local anaesthesia means a local loss of pain sensation.   T
3. Local anaesthetics have the advantage that:
    Patients remain conscious and usually mobile after the procedure.   T
    Hospitalisation is not always necessary.   T
    The patient can co-operate during the procedure.   T
    Fear of general anaesthesia is removed.   T
4. Examples of local anaesthetics include:
    Bipivucaine.   T
    Levobupivacaine.   T
    Lidocaine.   T
    Procaine.   T
    Ropivacaine.   T
5. Lidocaine is often formulated with ACh to constrict local vessels.   F
        Not ACh, but *epinephrine* to constrict vessels.
6. Local anaesthetics can be applied as gels.   T
7. Uses for topical application of local anaesthetics include:
    Perineal itching.   T
    Herpes infections.   T
    Epidural injections.   T
8. Adverse effects of local anaesthetics include:
    Hypertension.   F
      Hypotension.
    Bradycardia.   F
    Arrhythmias.   T
    Dangerous ventricular fibrillation.   T
    Asystole.   T
    Tinnitus.   T
    Seizures.   T
9. Local anaesthetics block Ca^{2+} channels on the axon membrane.   F
        Na^{2+} channels.

Chapter 35 Quiz answers

T = TRUE   F = FALSE

1. Premedication is used to dry secretions and allay anxiety.   T

2. Proton pump inhibitors may be used before surgery to reduce risk of acid respiration.   T
3. General anaesthetics are administered by inhalation or injection.   T
4. The ideal general anaesthetic:
   Has a narrow gap between Stages 3 and 4.   F
      Has as wide a margin as possible.
   Is non-flammable if a gas.   T
   Brings the patient slowly to Stage 3.   F
      Brings the patient rapidly to Stage 3.
   Does not impair cardiovascular or renal function.   T
   Abolishes appreciation of pain during surgery.   T
   Does not impair cardiovascular function.   T
   Has no hangover or after-effects.   T
5. There is a strong positive correlation between the MAC and the oil:gas partition coefficient.   F
      There is a strong *negative* correlation.
6. Halothane is associated with hepatotoxicity.   T
7. Ketamine can cause nightmares during recovery.   T
8. Thiopental can cause cardio-respiratory depression.   T
9. Suxamethonium is a non-depolarising muscle relaxant.   F
      Suxamethonium is a *depolarising* muscle relaxant.

Chapter 36 Quiz answers

T = TRUE   F = FALSE

1. Parkinson's disease:
   Is a degenerative disorder of the CNS.   T
   Usually presents between 50-65 years.   T
   Involves a progressive loss of sensory function.   F
      A progressive loss of motor, ANS and cognitive function.
   Is caused by degeneration of CNS noradrenergic neurones.   F
      A loss of nigrostriatal dopaminergic neurones.
2. Parkinson's disease is caused by unregulated firing of the cholinergic extrapyramidal system of the brain.   T
3. Drugs such MPTP can cause parkinsonian symptoms.   T
4. Parkinson's disease is treated with:
   Antimuscarinic drugs.   T
   Dopamine agonists.   T
   Monoamine oxidase-B inhibitors.   T
   COMT inhibitors.   T
5. Co-beneldopa is a mixture of levodopa and carbidopa.   F
      Levodopa and benserazide.

6. Adverse effects of levodopa include:
   Nausea and vomiting initially.   T
   Nightmares and hallucinations.   T
   Headaches.   T
   Dyskinesia.   T
   'On-off' phenomenon.   T
   Insomnia.   F
      'Sudden sleep' occurrence during the day.
7. Contraindications for levodopa include pregnancy, breast-feeding and
   closed-angle glaucoma.   T

Chapter 37 Quiz answers

T = TRUE   F = FALSE

1. Epilepsy:
   Is the occurrence of recurrent seizures.   T
   Is sometimes due to brain damage through trauma.   T
   May be idiopathic.   T
   May involve imbalances in glutaminergic/GABAergic systems.   T
   Can occur in children.   T
   Is usually by cerebella damage.   F
      More usually *cortical* damage.
2. Absence seizures may be typical or atypical.   T
3. Atypical seizures are prolonged.   T
4. Atypical seizures are usually caused by pre-existing neuronal damage.   T
5. Typical seizures are frequent, momentary episodes.   T
6. Drug treatment *may* be inappropriate if:
   There are no abnormal EEG changes.   T
   The patient had prolonged insomnia.   T
   There is no evidence of structural brain damage.   T
   The patient has a fever.   F
      The febrile patient should be considered for treatment.
7. The primary aim of drug therapy is to revive the patient.   F
      The primary aim of drug therapy is to prevent seizures.
8. Starting drugs for partial seizures include carbamazepine.   T
9. Gabapentin may be added as an adjunct drug for partial seizures.   T
10. Sodium valproate and topiramate have a risk of being teratogenic.   T
11. A family history of bone marrow depression is a contraindication for
    carbamazepine.   T
12. Patients on topiramate must be adequately hydrated.   T
13. General principles for drug treatment for generalised seizures include:
    Multiple drugs at first.   F

Monotherapy initially.

Increasing dose of first drug if ineffective.   T

Adequate supervision of patient compliance.   T

Monitoring for adverse effects, e.g. regular blood tests.   T

14. Phenytoin has the following disadvantages:

First order kinetics.   F

   Zero order kinetics.

High plasma protein binding.   T

Many drug interactions through, e.g. enzyme liver induction.   T

Adverse effects, e.g. gum hypertrophy.   T

15. Benzodiazepines are not associated with severe withdrawal problems.   F

   Adverse effects include sedation, dependence and seizure-producing withdrawal symptoms.

Chapter 39 Quiz answers

T = TRUE   F = FALSE

1. Depression may be caused by low monoaminergic brain activity.   T

2. MAOIs are the main drugs used to treat depression.   F

   MAOIs have been largely superseded by tricyclics and SSRIs.

3. SSRIs:

Prolong brain 5-HT activity by blocking re-uptake of 5-HT.   T

Include citalopram.   T

In young people may pose a suicide risk.   T

Are useful in the manic phase.   F

Should NOT be used in the manic phase.

4. Precautions for SSRIs include:

Diabetes.   T

Epilepsy.   T

Closed angle glaucoma.   T

5. Adverse effects of SSRIs include:

Withdrawal symptoms.   T

Diarrhoea.   T

Weight gain.   T

Abdominal cramps.   T

Hypersensitivity reactions.   T

6. MAOIs:

Are the mainstay of treatment for depression.   F

   No, largely superseded by SSRIs.

Include isocarbazid.   T

Are very dangerous with wine or cheese.   T

7. Tricyclic antidepressants inhibit re-uptake of 5-HT and NE.   T

8. Trimipramine is a tricyclic antidepressant.   T
9. Tricyclic antidepressants block acetylcholine reuptake.   F
    Tricyclics block norepinephrine and/or 5-HT reuptake.
10. Tricyclics are not recommended for panic attacks.   F
    Tricyclics may be used to treat panic attacks.
11. Tricyclics are indicated for moderate to severe depression with sleep
    disturbances.   T
12. ECT therapy may be needed initially when using tricyclics.   T
13. Tricyclics can cause paranoia as an adverse effect.   T
14. Tricyclics are contraindicated after a recent myocardial infarction.   T
15. Trazodone works by blocking MAO.   F
    Trazodone blocks 5-HT re-uptake and blocks 5-HT$_2$ receptors.

Chapter 40 Quiz answers

T = TRUE   F = FALSE

1. Clinical anxiety:
    Is characterised mainly by depression.   F
       More by fear and apprehension.
    Is a recurring problem for the patient.   T
    May bring on panic attacks.   T
    Symptoms include:
    Insomnia.   T
    Pessimism.   T
    Euphoria.   F
    Loss of libido.   T
    Hypochondria.   T
2. Drugs used include SSRIs.   T
3. Benzodiazepines are associated with severe withdrawal symptoms.   T
4. In elderly patients, benzodiazepines can produce amnesia and ataxia.   T
5. Benzodiazepines should not be prescribed for more than 4 months.   F
    Not more than 4 *weeks*.
6. Benzodiazepines are contraindicated with:
    Panic attacks.   T
    Sleep apnoea syndrome.   T
    Acute pulmonary insufficiency.   T
7. Compliance with drug regimes among anxious patients is often
    compromised because of adverse drug effects.   T

Chapter 41 Quiz answers

T = TRUE   F = FALSE

1.	Gram-negative bacteria stain red with crystal violet.	T
2.	Bateriostatic drugs do not kill the bacteria.	T
3.	Antibacterial drugs include:	
	Cephalosporins.	T
	Penicillins.	T
	Aminoglycosides.	T
	Sulphonamides.	T
	Macrolides.	T
4.	The choice of an antibacterial depends on:	
	The status of the patient.	T
	The site of the infection.	T
	The nature of the infective agent.	T
	The cellular or subcellular target.	T
	The patient's mental state.	F
5.	Bacterial resistance is failure of the drug to harm the infective organism.	T
6.	Bacterial resistance is caused by:	
	The patient's immune system.	F
	Resistance is due to bacterial mutation.	
	Incorrect use of the antibiotic.	T
	Feeding antibiotics to livestock.	T
	Incorrect diagnosis of the infecting organism.	T
	Over-prescribing.	T
7.	Bacterial adaptations to antibiotics include:	
	Increased capacity to degrade the antibiotic.	T
	Modification of the cell wall to exclude the drug.	T
	Cell wall mutation so the drug can't bind to it.	T
	Production of antibodies to the drug.	F
8.	Antiviral drugs:	
	Are used mainly for HIV and herpes.	T
	Include nucleoside reverse transcriptase inhibitors.	T
9.	Histoplasmosis is treated with abavacir.	F
	Histoplasmosis is a fungal infection; abavacir is antiviral.	
10.	Antifungal drugs include fluconazole.	T
11.	Artemether is used as prophylaxis in malaria.	F
	Artemether is used with benflumetol to treat *Falciparum* malaria.	
12.	Primaquine is prophylactic for malaria.	T
13.	Amoebic dysentery can be treated with metronidazole.	T
14.	Sand fly bites can cause Leishmaniasis.	T
15.	Leishmaniasis is treated with sodium stiboglutonate.	F
	Leishmaniasis is treated with Pyrimethamine + sulphadiazine.	

Chapter 42 Quiz answers

T = TRUE   F = FALSE

1.	Cytotoxic means poisonous to cells.	T
2.	Alkylating agents are highly specific in targeting cancer cells.	F
3.	Adverse effects of alkylating agents include:	
	Alopecia.	T
	Teratogenicity.	T
	Dementia.	F
	GIT disturbances.	T
	Bone marrow depression.	T
4.	Adverse effects of antimetabolites include:	
	Myelosuppression.	T
	Mucositis.	T
	Nausea and vomiting.	T
5.	Topoisomerase inhibitors stimulate DNA supercoiling.	F
	They *block* DNA supercoiling.	
6.	Antibiotics:	
	May act through the generation of free radicals.	T
	May act on enzymes.	T
7.	Estrogens exacerbate breast cancer.	T
8.	Antiestrogens block estrogen action.	T
9.	Tamoxifen is used for estrogen receptor-positive malignancy.	T
10.	Toremifene is indicated for premenopausal women.	F
	Postmenopausal women.	
11.	Bevacizumab is a monoclonal antibody stimulating blood vessel growth (angiogenesis).	F
	Bevacizumab *blocks* angiogenesis, thus inhibiting tumour growth.	
12.	Trastuzumab (Herceptin) is used for HER2-positive metastatic breast cancer.	T

Index